The
Infection
Prevention
HANDBOOK

Libby F. Chinnes, RN, BSN, CIC

+HCPro

The Infection Prevention Handbook is published by HCPro, Inc.

Copyright © 2009 HCPro, Inc.

ISBN: 978-1-60146-647-1

HCPro, Inc., provides information resources for the healthcare industry.

HCPro, Inc., is not affiliated in any way with The Joint Commission, which owns the JCAHO and Joint Commission trademarks.

Libby F. Chinnes, RN, BSN, CIC, Author
Tami Swartz, Editor
Owen MacDonald, Executive Editor
Emily Sheahan, Group Publisher
Susan Darbyshire, Cover Designer
Janell Lukac, Graphic Artist

Amanda Donaldson, Copyeditor
Amy Cohen, Proofreader
Matt Sharpe, Production Supervisor
Susan Darbyshire, Art Director
Jean St. Pierre, Director of Operations

HCPro, Inc.
P.O. Box 1168
Marblehead, MA 01945
Telephone: 800/650-6787 or 781/639-1872
Fax: 781/639-2982
E-mail: *customerservice@hcpro.com*

Visit HCPro at its World Wide Web sites:
www.hcpro.com and *www.hcmarketplace.com*

Contents

Your CD-ROM includes Appendix A: Sample Data Reports and Displays, which includes:

Appendix A Introduction

Figure A.1 Sample Quarterly Nosocomial Infection and Reportable Diseases Report

Figure A.2 Sample Infection Control Report on Obstetrician Unit

Figure A.3 Sample Infection Control Report to Performance Improvement Committee

Figure A.4 MRSA Tracking Log

Figure A.5 Sample Clostridium difficile Incident Report

Figure A.6 SICU Ventilator-Associated Pneumonias

Figure A.7 Sample MRSA Rate Per 1,000 Patient Days

Figure List

Figures are also included on the enclosed CD-ROM.

About the Author

Libby F. Chinnes, RN, BSN, CIC, has her own independent infection control consulting practice, IC Solutions, LLC, in Mt. Pleasant, SC. Chinnes has more than 25 years of experience in infection prevention and control and has been certified in the field since 1983. She provides consultation to infection control programs in assessment, problem solving, and training in acute care, long-term care, ambulatory care, home care, and long-term acute care and serves as a consultant to healthcare industries. Chinnes is a frequent speaker on infection prevention and control topics throughout the country.

CHAPTER 1
An Overview

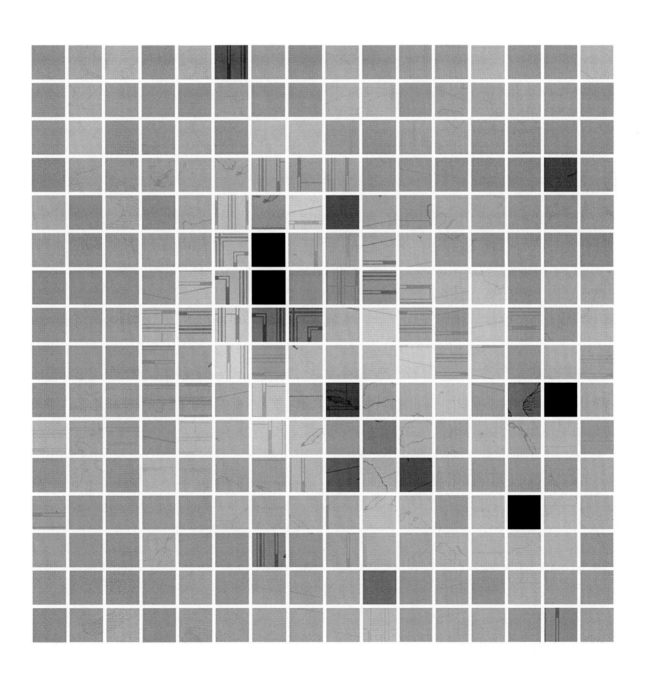

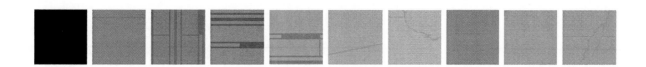

CHAPTER 1
An Overview

You have been given the position of infection preventionist (IP), also known as the infection prevention and control professional. It seems that once you leave your office for the nursing units or ancillary departments, everyone expects you to have all the answers. If you work in a small hospital or other facility such as long-term care or an ambulatory surgery center, you may even have other official duties such as employee health, staff development, or safety. The question becomes: Where do you start and how will you learn it all?

First, take a deep breath and realize that you do not have to have all the answers. You have plenty of resources available, including this book, training sessions, and other colleagues. Don't hesitate to reach out to them for answers. Second, remember that infection prevention and control is a specialty with much information to learn and, like any specialty, it will take time to become familiar with much of the literature and guidelines available.

ROLES AND RESPONSIBILITIES

First, let's discuss your new role as IP for your facility. A helpful reference is "APIC/CHICA-Canada Infection Prevention, Control, and Epidemiology: Professional and Practice Standards," available at *www.apic.org*.[1] The IP, whether just beginning or a seasoned professional, strives for competency in his or her role through education, certification, and incorporation of these standards into practice. The IP should periodically compare him- or herself and his or her program to these standards and use them as a guide.

Coordination of infection prevention and control program

The IP's role is to manage and coordinate infection prevention and control for the entire facility, or specific assigned areas, if working in a multiperson department under an infection prevention manager. The IP must ensure that proper infection prevention and control practices are followed in every department, including ancillary departments such as dietary, environmental services, pharmacy, and maintenance.

Development and maintenance of infection prevention and control policies and procedures

To this end, the facility must have infection prevention and control policies for every department as well as overall policies such as a bloodborne pathogens plan (exposure control plan) and a tuberculosis plan per the Occupational Safety and Health Administration. The IP does not have to write all these policies but should collaborate with department supervisors and advise on best infection prevention and control practice based on the most current guidelines, standards, and regulations. These policies and procedures should be on a schedule for review/revision in addition to those times when, for example, regulations change. Some of these policies and procedures are listed in Figure 1.1, and others may be added as needed or as new services arise.

FIGURE 1.1 • SAMPLE TABLE OF CONTENTS FOR INFECTION PREVENTION MANUAL

Section 1: General policies

1. Responsibilities, authority, and membership of the infection prevention and control committee (or applicable committee such as quality improvement if no infection prevention and control committee exists)
2. Responsibilities of the infection preventionist
3. Responsibilities of the hospital epidemiologist
4. Methods of surveillance
5. Definitions of healthcare-associated infections
6. Facility risk assessment
7. Facility infection control plan
8. Hand hygiene
9. Outbreak investigations
10. Standard precautions
11. Isolation techniques and requirements
12. Multidrug-resistant organism policy
13. Bloodborne pathogens exposure control plan
14. Tuberculosis control plan
15. Handling of sentinel events
16. Infectious wastes management
17. Influenza plan
18. Bioterrorism plan
19. Management of the influx or risk of influx of infectious patients (surge capacity)
20. Animals: service and therapy
21. Construction and renovation
22. Cleaning, storage, and distribution of patient care equipment
23. Refrigerator policy
24. Reporting of communicable diseases
25. Urinary tract infections prevention program
26. Ventilator-associated pneumonia prevention program
27. Bloodstream infections: catheter-associated prevention program

Section 2: Employees

1. Communicable disease exposures
2. Employee health policies

Section 3: Departmental policies

1. Biomedical engineering
2. Dietary/vending machines
3. Endoscopy
4. Engineering and facilities management
5. Environmental services
6. Hemodialysis
7. Imaging
8. Laboratory
9. Laundry
10. Materials management
11. Nursing
12. Pharmacy (multidosing and safe injection practices)
13. Physical therapy/occupational therapy/speech therapy
14. Respiratory therapy
15. Volunteers
16. OR
17. Decontamination, sterilization, and sterile processing

Surveillance and use of epidemiologic principles

Other roles of the IP are to perform surveillance of healthcare-associated infections per each facility's unique surveillance plan and inclusive of any mandatory surveillance as regulated by individual states. Surveillance is based on the population served, services offered, and previous surveillance data as well as high-risk, high-volume, and problem-prone events. For example, in a 250-bed hospital, a surveillance plan might entail:

- Coronary artery bypass surgery (high-volume procedure and mandated by certain states).

- Lumbar laminectomies (problem prone, as noted in past surveillance).

- Central line–associated bloodstream infections in ICUs and outside of ICUs (high risk and noted in The Joint Commission National Patient Safety Goals).

- Multidrug-resistant organisms (individual rates of methicillin-resistant *Staphylococcus aureus,* vancomycin-resistant *Enterococcus,* and extended-spectrum beta-lactamases). These are problem prone and mandated by certain states and The Joint Commission's National Patient Safety Goals. Also, *Clostridium difficile*, which is high risk and problem prone.

- Ventilator pneumonia in the surgical ICU.

- Influenza vaccine compliance of the staff.

- Compliance with hand hygiene and standard precautions by staff members, physicians, and all others (high risk, problem prone, and noted in the Joint Commission National Patient Safety Goals).

The IP should use epidemiological principles such as trending by time, person, and place and risk stratification to critically analyze surveillance data gathered, identify risk factors, and make recommendations for improvement based on those analyses. The IP must then give the data to those who need to know, such as patient care personnel, appropriate committees (e.g., infection control and critical care), and leadership in order to improve patient care. Surveillance is continued to determine whether the recommendations for improvement made a difference in patient care.

Education and training

One role that every IP is involved in is education and serving as a resource for providers, staff members, patients, and families on the most current scientific information in the infection prevention and control literature. By assessing the needs of his or her staff members, the IP uses the principles of adult learning to guide training in a variety of ways and separate fact from fiction.

Consulting

In the same light, IPs are the facility's internal consultants or experts on the most current guidelines, regulations, and standards on infection prevention and control. The field of infection prevention and control is constantly changing, and the IP is a valuable member of the healthcare team as an educator and facility consultant. The IP brings knowledge of basic infection prevention and control to all settings in the continuum of care, including acute, long-term, long-term acute, home care, and ambulatory care.

Employee health

IPs collaborate with the employee health department on strategies to decrease risk of infectious disease spread to patients from employees and to employees from patients. Strategies may include ensuring that proper immunizations are received, developing recommendations for healthcare worker restrictions for those with infectious conditions, and handling healthcare worker exposures to infectious diseases. In smaller facilities, the IP may also hold the role of the employee health professional and be accountable for fulfilling both job descriptions.

Performance improvement

IPs function as integral parts of performance improvement (PI) initiatives. In fact, it is often said that IPs were the first to practice PI before it was an established function. IPs may lead or be a member of a multidisciplinary performance improvement team.

Research

IPs also conduct, participate in, and evaluate research such as in surveillance findings, informal epidemiologic studies, and outbreaks. Much of the infection prevention and control research has been conducted in acute care settings. Although basic practices apply to all settings of care, more research is needed in alternative settings.

Program management, evaluation, and fiscal responsibility

To participate in all these roles, IPs must also manage the infection prevention and control program, which should be evaluated at least annually and more often as needed. Evaluation of the program includes determining whether goals and objectives were met and what needs to happen if they were unmet, while keeping financial responsibilities in mind.

Disaster preparedness

With the advent of bioterrorism, man-made disasters, and the threat of pandemics such as influenza, a fairly new role for the IP is also participation in the facility disaster preparedness program. IPs will be involved in all phases of a disaster including preparedness, impact, response, and recovery.

KEY PROFESSIONAL AND PERSONAL TRAITS

The IP is an experienced healthcare professional with a background in health sciences who strives to acquire and maintain competency in the dynamic field of infection prevention and control. The job is one in which learning never ceases. In fact, the IP appears to be a jack-of-all-trades, with knowledge in at least 16 content areas, which include:

- Epidemiology and outbreak management
- Infectious diseases
- Microbiology
- Patient care practices
- Asepsis
- Disinfection/sterilization
- Employee health
- Facility planning/construction
- Emergency preparedness
- Education principles
- Communication
- Evaluation of products
- Information technology
- Program administration
- Legislative issues
- Research

Don't be frightened by the long list of topics, as we all bring strengths to the table. You may have knowledge, education, and skills in infectious diseases yet need to learn much more about employee health and disinfection and sterilization. Whatever our weaknesses, we can gain the knowledge we need to succeed.

In addition to completing a basic course on infection prevention and control within the first six months of entering the field, the IP is encouraged to continuously read, attend training courses, and develop knowledge and skills in the areas listed above. One manner in which to demonstrate professional competency is to become certified and maintain certification through the Certification Board of Infection Control and Epidemiology. Many facilities advertise for experienced IPs who are certified in infection prevention and control.

Other personal traits of an IP that organizations look for when hiring are people skills, the ability to critically think through complex clinical scenarios, and a go-getting attitude. Solutions for infection prevention problems are often developed collaboratively with a team of multidisciplinary departments. For example, to deal with increased ventilator-associated pneumonia rates in the ICU, the IP may form a team composed of him- or herself, respiratory therapy staff members, critical care nursing staff members, and the medical director of the critical care unit. In another example, dealing with increased infection rates for *Clostridium difficile* housewide, the team may consist of the IP, clinical frontline nursing staff members, environmental services, and pharmacy. The IP must be able to work well with others whether on a daily basis on the nursing units and individual ancillary departments, at monthly/quarterly infection prevention and control committee meetings or performance improvement committees, or periodically to address issues with the chief operating officer (COO) or CEO. The IP must be able to influence diverse groups of people toward infection prevention and control. He or she is an index position to influence the quality of care provided to patients.

The IP may work as the sole practitioner in the infection prevention and control department, as the staff member under an experienced manager, or as the infection prevention manager in charge of other IPs. However, one person should be designated as responsible for the program. A hospital epidemiologist or infectious disease physician with infection control training may be available part-time or on a consultative basis to assist and guide the IP. Even though The Joint Commission no longer requires a specific infection control committee, some states do require one, and some organizations find that this is a crucial part of their program in that it gives administrative and political support to their efforts. Infection prevention is a critical function applicable to all departments and activities within the organization. It is really the responsibility of everyone who works within the organization. The IP at a small facility may even wear several hats in addition to this role, such as employee health coordinator, risk manager, or staff educator. Typically, the IP reports to the chief nursing officer, quality improvement director, or COO. Critical information from the infection prevention and control department must be taken all the way to the board of the hospital, for example, as well as shared with all departments and staff members.

There are many challenges and complexities for infection control. Emerging infectious diseases as well as the possibility of travel carrying these diseases to our individual doorsteps brings a sense of urgency and requires us to stay informed about current communicable diseases and world events. Working with all types and levels of staff members, and especially dealing with compliance with best patient care practices, is paramount. Networking, joining the Association for Professionals in Infection Control and Epidemiology, and staying abreast of current infection prevention literature will assist the creative IP in problem solving and helps prevent having to reinvent the wheel. In order to obtain an increase in salary, a promotion, additional staff members, or resources for the department, the IP must constantly demonstrate value not only in terms of clinical needs and patient satisfaction, but also cost. A program's effectiveness may be influenced greatly by the commitment of administration to infection prevention and control. In smaller facilities or nursing homes, for example, the IP may only be allowed a few hours per week to perform infection prevention activities. The IP must be granted the time and resources necessary to accomplish the program's goals.

IPs are mentors and leaders for best practice for patient safety. They are ethically oriented and professionally accountable in promoting patient and employee safety. Most IPs will tell you that serving as the patients' advocate is the role about which they are most passionate. There is no greater calling.

CONCLUSION

The IP performs a vital role for a healthcare facility and coordinates the infection prevention and control efforts of the entire organization. Through surveillance, development of sound policies and procedures (evidence-based and consistent with current regulations and standards), education, and performance improvement activities, the IP is able to influence safe care for patients and protection of employees. Although the role is complex, technical, ever-changing, and requires knowledge in many areas, the IP performs fulfilling work and serves as a champion for patient advocacy.

REFERENCES

1. C. Friedman, et al., "APIC/CHICA-Canada Infection Prevention, Control and Epidemiology: Professional and Practice Standards," *American Journal of Infection Control* 36 (2008): 385–389.

CHAPTER 2

Implementing and Organizing Your Infection Prevention and Control Program

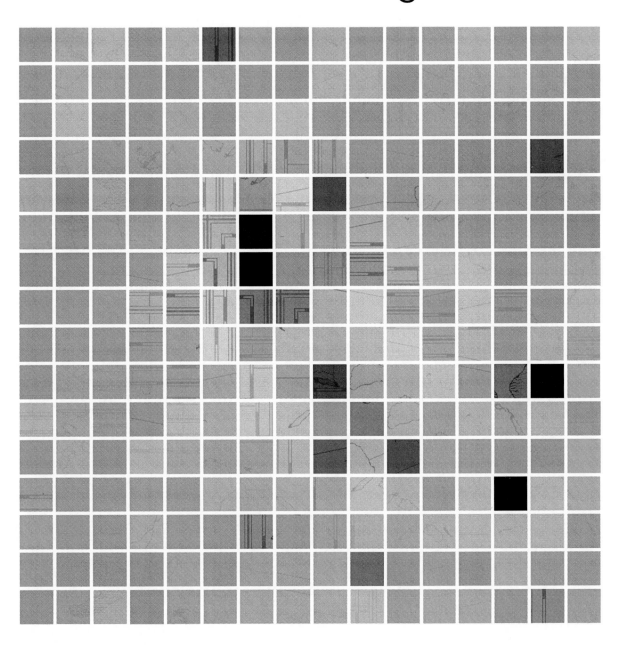

Implementing and Organizing Your Infection Prevention and Control Program

Whether the setting is acute, long-term, home health, or ambulatory care, every facility is required to have an active, coordinated, and effective infection control program. You may have inherited a well-established infection prevention and control program, or you may have to set one up from scratch. In either case, you need to know the broad tasks that need to be accomplished for patient safety and employee protection. Then you can begin to assess what works, and what needs some work!

INFRASTRUCTURE

The infection prevention and control program is usually under the direction of the infection prevention and control committee or other applicable committee, such as the quality performance or environment of care committee, both of which would report to the overall quality council and, ultimately, to the board of directors of the facility. All programs would benefit from the expertise of a staff or contracted hospital epidemiologist, or by having the ability to consult with someone with such expertise.[1] In addition to hospitals, all healthcare organizations should have ongoing access to the services of a person who is trained in infection prevention and control (i.e., an infection preventionist [IP]) and who provides oversight for the infection control program. The committee should also have access to the continuing services of a physician trained in healthcare epidemiology.[2] Joint Commission standards state that the committee and its designated representatives (i.e., the IP and the hospital epidemiologist) must have documented authority to institute preventive measures deemed appropriate for the prevention of healthcare-associated infections. This authority does not mean that the IP and epidemiologist could close a unit during an influenza outbreak; however, it does mean they would consult with the clinical and administrative leaders and guide the facility's decision for the safety of all patients and employees.

At many facilities, especially smaller ones, there is only one IP, who might wear multiple hats and serve as an employee health professional, a staff nurse, or in other roles. The *SHEA/APIC Guideline: Infection Prevention and Control in the Long-Term Care Facility*[3] notes that an oversight committee, typically a small group consisting of the administrator, the IP, and the medical director, has formal delegation of infection control program oversight. It also says that consultation with an infectious disease physician or other professional with infection control expertise should be made. The IP should be responsible for directing the activities of the infection prevention and control program and have written authority to institute emergency infection control measures and sufficient knowledge, time, and administrative support to direct the program.

It's also critical to note that in some facilities, such as an ambulatory surgery center, the IP may also work part-time as a perioperative professional, and there may be no epidemiologist available for consultation. Many outbreaks have occurred in nonhospital settings in recent years. Therefore, it is important for these settings to have access to a trained IP who has oversight of the infection prevention and control program.

STAFFING

According to the Delphi Project,[4] 0.8 to one IP for every 100 occupied acute care beds is recommended. This ratio is usually not met, especially when the IP has to cover alternative settings as part of the system. For example, as part of his or her responsibility, the IP may cover a 250-bed acute care hospital, a 20-bed long-term care unit, plus 30 physician offices. Or the IP in long-term care may have only a few hours per week to devote to infection prevention and control and yet may still be responsible for employee health and supervising nursing staff members. Although *SHEA/APIC Guideline: Infection Prevention and Control in Long-Term Care Facility* makes no recommendation on the number of IPs per 100 long-term care facility beds; however Canadian infection control experts have voiced the need for one full-time, formally trained IP per 150–250 long-term beds.[5] The acuity of patients, risks of the population, and complexity of the healthcare system must be taken into consideration for infection prevention and control staffing.

If you are lucky enough to have more than one IP, one person should be assigned responsibility and accountability for the overall program, usually the more experienced IP. Duties may be divided by tasks, nursing units, or service lines. For example, two IPs may divide the nursing units and departments, or one may be responsible for two surveillance initiatives housewide, ongoing employee infection prevention and control education, and two-thirds of the hospital departments and the other has an additional three surveillance initiatives, new employee orientation, and the remaining one-third of the departments for review of practices and revision of policies and procedures.

Two Society for Healthcare Epidemiology of America (SHEA) reports address requirements for infection prevention and control programs in the hospital setting and out-of-hospital setting. They are:

- "Requirements for Infrastructure and Essential Activities of Infection Control and Epidemiology in Hospitals: A Consensus Panel Report and Requirements for Infrastructure"[6]

- "Requirements for Infrastructure and Essential Activities of Infection Control and Epidemiology Activities in Out-of-Hospital Settings"[7]

According to the first SHEA report on hospital settings, "all hospitals should have the continuing services of a trained hospital epidemiologist(s) and ICP(s). Category I recommendation."[8] (See

Figure 2.1 for and explanation of SHEA recommendations and category descriptions). The epidemiologist may be full-time, part-time, or a contracted consultant. In the second SHEA report on out-of-hospital settings, it is stated that "all HCOs [healthcare organizations] should have access to the ongoing services of a person who is trained in infection prevention and control (i.e., an infection control professional), who provides oversight for the infection control program. Category II," and "All HCOs should have access to continuing services of a physician trained in healthcare epidemiology. Category II."[9] Certification in the field is highly encouraged.

FIGURE 2.1 • SHEA RECOMMENDATIONS[10]

I. Strongly recommended for implementation based on evidence from one of the following:

- At least one properly randomized, controlled trial

- At least one well-designed clinical trial without randomization

- Cohort or case-control analytical studies (preferably from more than one center)

- Multiple time-series studies

II. Recommended for implementation based on one of the following:

- Published clinical experience or descriptive studies

- Reports of expert committees

- Opinions of respected authorities

III. Recommended when required by government rules or regulations (see articles for specific categories of recommendations)

In uncertain economic times, all IPs need to learn to work smarter and not harder. (See "Tips for the busy IP" later in this chapter.) Many IPs working alone have implemented the concept of infection prevention and control liaisons. These are staff members on each unit or department who have a keen interest in infection prevention and who can be trained to be the "mini IP" on the unit. They can be taught to perform such tasks as data collection, compliance monitoring, education, peer immunization, tuberculin skin test readings, and environmental rounds, among other duties. The IP should maintain ongoing training for the liaisons on a regular basis, such as quarterly. Another tip for the busy IP is to manage interruptions. For example, block off two hours of uninterrupted office time on your calendar for analysis of surveillance data and reports. Only answer emergency phone calls, and do not check your e-mail during this time.

TIPS FOR THE BUSY IP
- Plan
- Prioritize
- Partner
- Identify a champion
- Divide tasks
- Delegate
- Simplify
- Standardize
- Manage interruptions
- Get rid of time wasters
- Handle paper efficiently (with labels such as trash, read, act on, and file)
- Go electronic when possible
- Use infection prevention and control liaisons
- Don't reinvent the wheel

Clerical assistance can also provide a tremendous advantage to your program; however, many programs do not have the services of a secretary, and the IP may have to use such creative tactics as sharing clerical help with another department, bartering for clerical help, or relying on a trained volunteer to provide these services.

RESOURCES

Who can you turn to for help? Your IP colleagues in the facility and your local community are wonderful resources. You should join a local chapter of the Association for Professionals in Infection Control and Epidemiology (APIC), as well as the national organization. The friends and colleagues you meet through this organization and through your training will be glad to mentor you and answer questions. Also, by attending meetings of this association and remaining current with infection prevention and control literature, you will begin to learn the many practical ways in which to develop workable forms, checklists, and solutions. Most are happy to share their knowledge and resources with you. If you have a hospital epidemiologist or infectious disease physician available, they are usually members of SHEA and will bring valuable input to infection control issues. As the IP, you may also want to join SHEA and participate in its training. APIC has basic, intermediate, and advanced educational offerings for IPs and provides education in many forms, such as free Webinars, elimination guides for certain diseases, patient education brochures, manuals, reference books, and other items. APIC also provides references for practicing infection control for many settings, such as long-term care, home care, ambulatory care, and behavioral health, as well as a must-have *APIC Text of Infection Control and Epidemiology*, a daily resource for any IP. APIC and SHEA both produce monthly journals, *American Journal of Infection Control* and *Infection Control and Hospital Epidemiology*, available free to their members or for purchase to nonmembers.

Don't forget about developing and maintaining partners throughout the organization. Perioperative nurses may assist the IP in feeling comfortable behind the closed doors of the operating room and in teaching him or her to recognize noncompliance with proper technique. Most critical care nurses are happy to share their knowledge and expertise with us on the newest technologies and invasive procedures. The dietary manager usually knows food regulations by heart and can assist us in the area of food safety. For microbiology, technologists can help us become more proficient in understanding ordered tests and the organisms that cause patients' problems.

As you can see, infection prevention is all about building relationships. We need to forge many new partnerships to help us achieve success in our programs. And last, but certainly not least, we need the support of committed, top-level leaders to assist us in reaching our goals for patient safety and employee health. This includes support of ongoing professional education for the IP and hospital epidemiologist. Without this major arm of support, it is very difficult to run a successful program.

RISK ASSESSMENT

According to The Joint Commission, a facility must first identify its risks for acquiring and transmitting infections. Once the risks are identified, then goals for the program can be developed. Per The Joint Commission, risks should be based on geographic location, community, and population served; care, treatment, and services provided; and analysis of surveillance data.

The risk assessment is not conducted solely by the IP; rather, a multidisciplinary group including at least infection prevention and control, the medical staff, nursing, and leadership must help to identify and evaluate risks. Then the IP will be able to document and prioritize risks. The entire infection prevention and control program of the facility is based on this important risk assessment. The risk assessment should be reviewed at least annually and whenever significant change occurs. For example, if the facility began to perform bronchoscopes on patients, a new service and level of risk has been added. The training of staff members for competencies and care, cleaning, and high-level disinfection of the bronchoscope is critical. Therefore, at this time, the risk assessment should be evaluated and revised again.

GOALS AND FUNCTIONS OF THE PROGRAM

"The overall goals of infection programs in hospitals and out-of-hospital settings are to:

- Protect patients from infection

- Protect healthcare workers, visitors, and others in the healthcare environment

- Implement the first two goals in a timely, efficient, and cost-effective manner, when possible"[11]

A program's more specific goals and objectives should fall under the overall goals. For example, one facility's goal may be to decrease central line–associated bloodstream infections. But to reach that goal, the IP needs to document in his or her infection control plan a very specific and measurable objective such as "decreased central line–associated bloodstream infections in all of ICUs by 25% in the next quarter." By documenting measurable objectives, the IP can then determine whether goals were successfully met or, if not, whether additional strategies for improvement are necessary. Another goal might be to increase awareness/compliance of influenza vaccine among healthcare workers. A measurable objective for this goal might be to increase influenza vaccine compliance systemwide by 20% during the next influenza season.

Goals should be based on the risk assessment of the organization and prioritized. By noting the goals in the written infection control plan for the facility, the IP has a documented road map to follow to improve outcomes at this particular setting. Also, the entire infection control plan should be taken to committee for approval at least annually. It is important to have the support of leadership for the infection control plan. The goals should be realistic and routinely tracked. This information should be part of the performance improvement program of the facility. The goals, objectives, and plan should be evaluated at least annually, and also whenever risks change.

Program functions

According to the SHEA reports, the principle functions of the program are to:

- "Obtain and manage critical data and information, including surveillance for infections

- Develop and recommend policies and procedures

- Intervene directly to prevent infections

- Educate and train healthcare workers, providers, patients, and nonmedical caregivers"[12]

More functions may be added to each unique program, such as construction and renovation consultation, evaluation of new products, and participation in performance improvement activities and committees, such as safety. Recommendations in the SHEA reports were rated according to the strength of the evidence in the literature. See Figure 2.1 earlier in this chapter.

According to these sources, surveillance of HAI infections must be performed, analyzed, and used to improve outcomes.

SURVEILLANCE

Surveillance is the cornerstone of infection control interventions. Through surveillance, the IP identifies and describes events to be studied. The IP also defines the population at risk (the denominator in the IP surveillance formula). The IP must select appropriate measurement, including risk stratification. Data sources need to be identified as well as personnel and methods to collect data. Numerators and denominators must actually be defined. By reporting the surveillance data back as meaningful information to staff members and providers, the IP can make them aware of issues such as an increase in ventilator-associated pneumonia or employee needlestick rates and the need to address them with best practices.

Specific events to be monitored should be based on individual state regulations regarding mandatory reporting, validated national benchmarks adjusted for patient risk, and the organization's strategic plan. This surveillance plan can be documented in the written infection prevention and control management plan for the facility. See Chapter 6 for more information.

The IP must also recommend scientifically valid infection control policies and procedures that are documented, implemented, and revised periodically. Policies usually are readily available in the infection control manual and revised periodically as needed (e.g., the bloodborne pathogens policy is revised annually as required by the Occupational Safety and Health Administration [OSHA]).

These policies should be based on current infection control guidelines and literature, practicality, and cost and should comply with regulations and accreditation requirements. A new employee or the IP should be able to read and understand the organization's specific policies and procedures that will guide their practice. Periodic monitoring of these policies and procedures should also be performed. Compliance is always an issue, as we are dealing with humans. We'll cover this more in Chapter 7. Policies and procedures should lead to improved prevention or patient outcomes. One of the policies should relate to required reporting of communicable diseases to the health department. This list is updated annually by the health department. In out-of-hospital settings as well as hospital settings, it is recommended that IPs develop policies and procedures for ongoing communication with other healthcare facilities as patients move between the systems and report any infections or adverse outcomes to the organization where the procedure was performed or from which the patient was discharged. They should also report epidemiological-significant organisms to the facility to which the patient will be transferred (for an example of this report, see Figure 2.2) For example, an IP who works for a group of physician offices may find that a patient has an infection at the harvest site after a coronary artery bypass procedure was performed. The IP would report this to the hospital where the heart surgery was done so it can count the occurrence in its statistics.

FIGURE 2.2 • SAMPLE FORM—NOTIFICATION OF INFECTION TO OUTSIDE FACILITIES									
Sent Notification	Received Notification	Patient's Name	MR#	Room	Date (Admit/ Discharge)	Facility	Condition/ Organism	Name of Contact	Comments

Source: Reprinted with permission from Barbara Russell.

One of the crucial areas in an organization's policy and procedure manual is employee health. The IP should collaborate with the employee health department and approve all policies and procedures in that area that relate to transmission of infection. This should include at-hire recommendations for employees as well as periodic medical evaluations. Employees must be offered appropriate immunizations and tuberculin skin tests, and there should be protocols for handling employee exposures to infectious diseases as well as indications for work restrictions, all of which should be based on Centers for Disease Control and Prevention (CDC) guidelines, regulations such as those from OSHA and state health departments, and weekly updates in *Morbidity and Mortality,* a CDC publication.

To be able to prevent diseases from spreading, all facilities must have the capacity to identify clusters or outbreaks of infectious diseases. The IP should review microbiology records regularly to identify clusters of unusual organisms or incidence of certain strains that are greater than usual. By performing surveillance and conducting rounds to all units and departments throughout the facility, the IP can maintain contact with frontline staff members for knowledge of disease clusters and can also monitor infection control practices in addition to providing consultation. The IP must have written authority and adequate resources to intervene with measures, such as audits of practice and education, as well as to conduct outbreak investigations.

Last, trained IPs must actively plan and provide ongoing educational programs for healthcare workers on infection prevention and control. These programs may include current infectious disease trends, prevention strategies, and the organization's surveillance data and recommendations. Programs should take into consideration the audience involved and should be evaluated for effectiveness. Don't forget training for the night and weekend staff, contracted staff, licensed independent professionals, students, and volunteers. In the *Infection Control and Hospital Epidemiology* report on out-of-hospital settings[13] as well as in the Joint Commission standards, it is recommended that organizations have a mechanism to ensure that patients and caregivers receive appropriate information regarding infection prevention and control as well.

Making your infection prevention and control efforts part of the overall performance improvement program for the organization can lead to improved patient outcomes and employee safety through:

- Monitoring of compliance with policies and procedures
- Reporting of meaningful data

- Education of staff members and patients on findings and basic principle of infection prevention

- Interventions based on best practice

- Continued surveillance to determine whether problems were corrected

CONCLUSION

Along with good infrastructure and staffing for infection prevention and control, the IP can meet goals and specific objectives of the program through four basic functions: surveillance, policies and procedures, interventions, and education of healthcare workers and patients. By following the basic organization of infection prevention and control programs in the two references noted, the IP can develop and improve a program in any setting.

REFERENCES

1. W. E. Scheckler, et al., "Requirements for Infrastructure and Essential Activities of Infection Control and Epidemiology in Hospitals: A Consensus Panel Report," *Infection Control and Hospital Epidemiology* 19.1 (1998): 114–124.

2. C. Friedman, et al., "Requirements for Infrastructure and Essential Activities of Infection Control and Epidemiology in Out-of-Hospital Settings: A Consensus Panel Report," *Infection Control and Hospital Epidemiology* 27.5 (1999): 418–429.

3. Phillip W. Smith, et al., "SHEA/APIC Guideline: Infection Prevention and Control in the Long-Term Care Facility," *American Journal of Infection Control* 36 (2008): 504–535.

4. C. O'Boyle, M. Jackson, S. J. Henly, "Staffing Requirements for Infection Control Programs in U.S. Health Care Facilities: Delphi Project," *American Journal of Infection Control* 30.6 (2002): 321–333.

5. J. Morrison, "Development of a Resource Model for Infection Prevention and Control Programs in Acute, Long-Term, and Homecare Settings: Conference Proceedings of the Infection Prevention and Control Alliance," *American Journal of Infection Control* 32 (2004): 2–6.

6. Scheckler, et al.

7. Friedman, et al.

8. Scheckler, et al.

9. Friedman, et al.

10. Scheckler, et al.

11. Ibid.

12. Ibid.

13. Friedman, et al.

The Four Major Sites of Infection

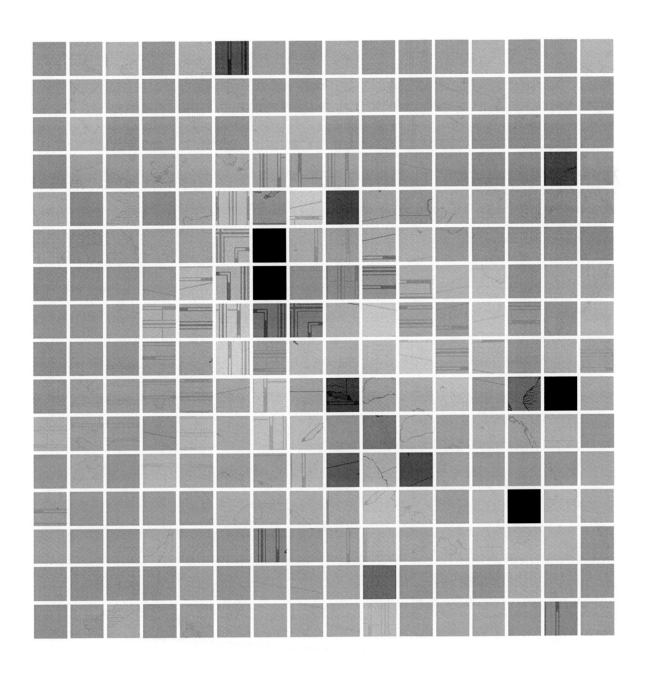

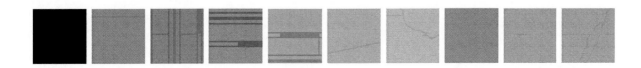

The Four Major Sites of Infection

One of the basic functions of any infection prevention and control program is surveillance of healthcare-associated infections. Although the infection preventionist (IP) may survey all sites of infection, targeted surveillance by site may be more efficacious because of known interventions that can be implemented to reduce many of these infections. Today's healthcare systems have scarce resources and many are subject to mandatory state public reporting of healthcare-associated infections. These two facts most likely lead the IP to focus on healthcare-associated infections at four major sites:

- Urinary tract (catheter-associated)

- Pneumonia (ventilator-associated)

- Bloodstream infection (central line-associated)

- Surgical site infection (SSI)

A discussion of each of the four sites follows along with risk factors and strategies for prevention.

The Institute of Healthcare Improvement has great "How-To Guides" on their Web site addressing all these major sites of infection (*www.ihi.org*).

URINARY TRACT INFECTIONS

Urinary tract infections (UTI) are the most common type of healthcare-associated infections.[1] Each year, they contribute substantially to increased morbidity, mortality, and cost. In the acute care setting, most UTIs are due to urinary instrumentation, such as indwelling bladder catheters, suprapubic catheters, and intermittent catheterization. The *APIC Text of Infection Control and Epidemiology*[2] lists the methods of introduction of organisms into the bladder.

Many different pathogens cause catheter-associated UTIs. Besides *E. coli* and yeasts, which were the most common in hospitals between 2006 and 2007, according to The Centers for Disease Control and Prevention's (CDC) National Healthcare Safety Network, other organisms include *Enterococcus, Pseudomonas aeruginosa, Klebsiella pneumonia*, and *Enterobacter, Staphylococcus* and other gram-negative bacteria.[3] Patients may acquire catheter-associated UTIs (CAUTI) in all settings across the continuum of care.

Patients may either be colonized (i.e., with no signs and symptoms of infection) or actually infected. CAUTIs may lead to urosepsis or bloodstream infection from infection in the urinary tract. UTIs—the majority of which are catheter-related—are the most common cause of bacteremias.[4] Many CAUTIs may be preventable with recommended infection control practices. In fact, The Centers for Medicare & Medicaid Services (CMS), which in the past paid for patient services without regard to outcome, now considers CAUTIs as a "never event." As of October 1, 2008, CMS will not reimburse for CAUTIs that were not present on admission in inpatients later discharged from acute care hospitals. Many UTIs are catheter-associated, asymptomatic, and need no treatment; however, they can also contribute to the morbidity and mortality rates and increased cost.

Risk factors

Most UTIs are catheter-associated in the acute care setting. The risk of UTI is directly proportional to the catheter duration, which is why it is of critical importance to remove the catheter as soon as possible.

Bacteria may enter the bladder in three ways. First, bacteria may ascend into the urinary tract through insertion of the catheter into the meatus, along the external (extraluminal) surface of the catheter. If this occurs early after catheter insertion, it suggests a lack of asepsis at insertion of the catheter. Second, microorganisms may move along the external catheter surface across the catheter-urethra interface to the bladder. Introduction of bacteria with catheter use is often associated with catheter-related biofilms. These biofilms often serve as the primary means in the development of CAUTIs. Once a biofilm is developed, the only way to eliminate the risk of a CAUTI is to remove the catheter. Third, microbes may ascend to the bladder by opening the otherwise closed system and by reflux up the catheter lumen from contaminated tubing and collection bag.

In The Society for Healthcare Epidemiology of America (SHEA) and The Infectious Diseases Society of America's (IDSA) report, *Strategies to Prevent Catheter-Associated Urinary Tract Infections in Acute Care Hospitals: A Compendium of Strategies to Prevent Healthcare Associated Infections in Acute Care Hospitals,*[5] the most important risk factor for development of CAUTI is the duration of catheterization. Additional risk factors were noted to be female sex, older age, and not maintaining a closed drainage system.

Prevention and control of UTIs

One of the most effective methods of UTI prevention is avoiding the use of an indwelling catheter or discontinuing its use when it is no longer indicated. Consider legitimate indications for catheterization in the first place and documenting the indication in the medical record. Indications for catheterization include:

- Perioperative use for selected surgeries

- Management of acute urinary retention and obstruction

- At patient request for comfort (exception)[6]

Indwelling catheters should not be used to replace nursing care for incontinent patients or to obtain urine for culture or tests when the patient can void voluntarily. Indwelling catheters should not be used for prolonged periods postoperatively without appropriate indications, or routinely for patients receiving epidural anesthesia/analgesia. Alternatives to indwelling catheterization should be evaluated, such as the condom catheter or intermittent catherization.[7] Catheters should only be inserted or manipulated with the use of sterile techniques by competent staff members, families, or patients. The smallest catheter possible should be used along with a sterile lubricant. Catheters placed in emergencies should be changed or removed as soon as possible.

The SHEA/IDSA *Compendium* goes on to recommend basic practices for ALL acute care hospitals to prevent and monitor CAUTIs. What follows is a summary of these basic practices. Organizations must implement written guidelines for use, insertion, and maintenance of catheters.

Use of indwelling urethral catheters should be limited to the following situations: perioperative use for selected surgeries, monitoring urinary output in critically ill, managing acute urinary retention and obstruction, assisting incontinent residents with pressure ulcer healing, and as an exception, to improve comfort per patient request.

As noted earlier, catheters should be inserted only when necessary for care and left in place only as long as indications remain. As part of an organization's quality improvement efforts, appropriate use of catheters as well as a system of daily rounds or reminders for daily assessment of continued catheter use may be very helpful. Only trained personnel should insert and maintain urinary catheters with the use of aseptic technique. Indications for insertion, date/time of insertion, individual inserting catheter, and date/time of catheter removal should be documented in the patient record. Other methods such as condom catheters or in-and-out catheters should be considered when appropriate.

As with all patient care, hand hygiene is paramount. Hand hygiene should be practiced immediately before insertion of the catheter and before/after manipulation of the catheter or apparatus. For the insertion, gloves, drape, sponges, sterile or antiseptic solution for cleaning the urethral meatus, and sterile lubricant jelly for insertion (single use) should be used. The smallest catheter possible should be used to minimize trauma.

Indwelling catheters should be properly secured after insertion and maintained with unobstructed urine flow and collecting bag below the level of bladder. A sterile, continuously closed drainage system must be maintained. The catheter and drainage tube should not be disconnected unless the catheter must be irrigated. There is no arbitrary time to change the catheter or the bag. The collecting system should be replaced with use of aseptic technique and after disinfecting the catheter tubing junction when breaks in aseptic technique, disconnection, or leakage occur. Small samples of urine for specimens may be aspirated from the sampling port with a sterile needle and syringe after cleansing the port with a disinfectant. The specimen should be transported promptly to the lab for culture.

Urine cultures should not be obtained from asymptomatic patients as an inappropriate treatment may result, which may lead to antimicrobial resistance as well as avoidable adverse effects. Larger volumes of urine may be aseptically obtained from the drainage bag. The drainage bag should be emptied regularly, using a separate collection container per patient. The draining spigot should not be allowed to touch the collecting drainage container or the floor. Routine hygiene is appropriate and cleaning the meatal area with an antiseptic is unnecessary.

In addition, surveillance of CAUTI must be conducted on the basis of the facility's risk assessment. Such surveillance should take into consideration frequency of catheter usage and potential risk factors such as type of surgery, obstetrics, and critical care. Standardized surveillance definitions should be used to identify patients with CAUTI. Catheter days should be collected for all patients and the groups or units being monitored. Measurements for surveillance purposes include:

- CAUTI rates for target populations
- Percentage of patients with indwelling catheter or inserted during hospitalization
- Percentage of acceptable catheter use indications
- Duration of indwelling catheter usage

Lastly, accountability plays a huge role in prevention of CAUTI from the CEO and senior management to front-line staff members at the bedside. Infection prevention is everyone's responsibility.

Of note are "special approaches" for the prevention of CAUTI, which are also included in The SHEA/IDSA *Compendium*. Refer to this SHEA/IDSA document for discussion of the special approaches. These special approaches are to be used when data and/or risk assessment suggests lack of effective control despite use of basic practices. They include:

- Perform a CAUTI risk assessment
- Identify and remove catheters no longer necessary organizationwide by one or more of the following methods: daily review of necessity of the catheter, chart or electronic reminders, such as automatic stop order requiring renewal or standardized reminders in the chart or electronic record, or daily unit rounds by nursing and physicians to review continuing necessity for catheters
- Develop postop management protocol for urinary retention, including use of intermittent catheterization and bladder scans by trained nurses
- Analyze and report use of catheters and adverse events from catheters such as CAUTI, obstruction, unintended removal, catheter trauma, or reinsertion after 24 hours of removal

Catheter insertion

Catheters should only be inserted or manipulated with the use of sterile techniques by competent staff members, families, or patients. Hand hygiene should be performed immediately before and after catheter manipulation. The meatus should be cleaned with an antiseptic before catheter insertion. Once the catheter is inserted aseptically, it should be secured properly. Urinary flow should be unobstructed. The urine collection bag should always remain below the level of the bladder whether the patient is ambulatory or in bed or a wheelchair.

When emptying the bag, ensure that the spigot does not contact the container and cross contaminate. Each patient should have his or her own collection container for emptying the collection bag regularly.

Catheter maintenance[8]

The patient should be bathed daily around the catheter as part of the bath or after a bowel movement. No other arbitrary routine cleansing around the catheter is needed.

Catheter irrigation should be avoided; however, if irrigation must be performed, the catheter-tubing junction should be disinfected before disconnection and flushing with a sterile system and irrigant. If frequent irrigation is required, the catheter should be changed.

Catheters placed in emergencies should be changed or removed as soon as possible. When breaches in technique, disconnection, or leakage occur, replace the collection system using the aseptic technique and after disinfecting the catheter-tubing junction.

There is no routine time interval to change a catheter. However, catheters should be left in place only as long as necessary.

Maintain a closed drainage system. When a urine specimen is needed, obtain a sample aseptically through the sampling port after disinfection of the port. Patients with UTIs should not share the same room or adjacent beds with noninfected patients.

When emptying the bag, ensure that the spigot does not contact the container and cross contaminate. Each patient should have his or her own collection container for emptying the collection bag regularly.

A 'bundle' approach to prevention

A bundle is a series of evidence-based interventions that, when applied simultaneously, have demonstrated a decrease in infection rates. An example of a bladder bundle, shown in APIC's *Guide to the Elimination of Catheter-Associated Urinary Tract Infections* (2008) is given below:

BLADDER BUNDLE INTERVENTIONS

- Aseptic insertion and proper maintenance is paramount
- Bladder ultrasound may avoid indwelling catheterization
- Use condom or intermittent catheterization in appropriate patients
- Do not use the indwelling catheter unless you must
- Ensure early removal of the catheter using reminders or stop orders[9]

The following are recommended strategies from APIC's *Guide to Elimination of Catheter-Associated Urinary Tract Infections* (2008) to prevent CAUTIs:

- "Adequately assess and document the need for urinary catheters based on recognized indications
- Use catheters in operative patients only as necessary
- Use the UTI prevention bundle
- Remove urinary catheters as soon as possible (for operative patients who have an indication for a catheter, preferably remove within 24 hours)
- Implement systems to alert care providers to evaluate the necessity for urinary catheters on a daily basis
- Do not use catheters in patients and nursing home patients for management of incontinence
- Provide regular feedback to staff members on process and/or outcome measures
- Implement quality improvement programs to reduce catheter use and the risk of UTIs"[10]

PNEUMONIA

Pneumonia is the second most common healthcare-acquired infection (HAI)[11] but is accompanied by the highest morbidity and mortality rate (15%-50%, according to APIC's *Guide to the Elimination of Ventilator-Associated Pneumonia*[12] [2009]). Pneumonia is an inflammation of the lungs that can present as community-acquired pneumonia (CAP) (i.e., pneumonia not associated with healthcare) or healthcare-associated pneumonia (HAP), which occurs 48 hours or more after admission to a healthcare facility. Much of HAP is ventilator-associated pneumonia (VAP), as the incidence of HAP increases dramatically when the patient is mechanically ventilated (six- to 20-fold).[13]

VAP is one of the most common infections that adults and children acquire in ICUs.[14] The most common cause of CAP or HAP is aspiration of oropharyngeal flora. The three most common manners in which VAP develops are aspiration, colonization of the aerodigestive tract, and use of contaminated equipment. The literature suggests, however, that many VAPs could be prevented by addressing the process of care.

Risk factors

The SHEA/IDSA *Compendium* notes risk factors for VAP to include:

- Prolonged intubation

- Enteral feeding

- Witnessed aspiration

- Paralytic agents

- Underlying illness

- Extremes of age

Other risk factors may include smoking, thoracic surgery, upper abdominal surgery, depressed level of consciousness, oral or nasogastric tubes, frequent ventilator circuit changes, and exposure to contaminated equipment or medications. Some patients may have multiple risk factors.

Common etiologic agents of pneumonia[15]

Pneumonia may be caused by the following microorganisms:

- **CAP:** *Streptococcus* pneumonia, H. influenza, *Mycoplasma* pneumonia, *Chlamydia* pneumonia, *Streptococcus Staphylococcus aureus*, *Streptococcus pyogenes*, *Klebsiella* pneumonia, and other Gram-negatives such as *Legionella,* influenza, and others

- **Early onset HAP** (within four to six days of admission to the hospital): *Streptococcus* pneumonia, H. influenza, *Moraxella catarrhalis, Staphylococcus aureus, E. coli, Proteus, Klebsiella,* and other Gram-negatives

- **Late onset HAP** (seven days or more in the hospital): *Streptococcus* pneumonia, H. influenza, *Moraxella catarrhalis, Staphylococcus aureus, E. coli, Proteus, Klebsiella,* and other Gram-negatives, *Pseudomonas aeruginosa, Enterobacter, Acinetobacter,* methicillin-resistant *Staphylococcus aureus,* and, rarely, anaerobes and fungi

In many cases, the cause of pneumonia is never determined.

Prevention and control of pneumonia

General strategies for prevention from the SHEA/IDSA *Compendium* include surveillance for VAP, hand hygiene, use of noninvasive ventilation when possible, minimization of the duration of ventilation, performance of daily readiness to wean assessments and use of weaning protocols, and education of healthcare workers about VAP. Other SHEA/IDSA "Compendium" interventions to prevent VAP are aimed at the three most common mechanisms by which VAP develops:

- Prevention of aspiration:

  - Unless contraindicated, elevate head of bed 30°–45°

  - Avoid gastric over distention

  - Avoid unplanned extubation and reintubation

  - Use a cuffed endotracheal tube (ET) with in-line or subglottic suctioning

  - Maintain an ET cuff pressure of at least 20 cm H_2O

- Interventions to reduce colonization of the aerodigestive tract:

  - Orotracheal incubation is preferred as nasotracheal increases risk of sinusitis and may increase risk of VAP

  - Histamine 2–receptor blocking agents and proton pump inhibitors for patients not at high risk of developing a stress ulcer or gastritis should be avoided (considered an unresolved issue by Healthcare Infection Control)

  - Healthcare Infection Control Practices Advisory Committee guidelines as well as use of sucralfate

  - Oral care should be performed with an antiseptic (frequency unresolved)

- Interventions to minimize contamination of equipment used with mechanical ventilation:

  - Reusable respiratory equipment should be rinsed with sterile water

  - Condensate should be removed from ventilator circuits while keeping the circuit closed

  - Ventilator circuit should be changed only when visibly soiled or malfunctioning

  - Respiratory therapy equipment should be stored and disinfected properly

In addition, all patients at risk of pneumonia should be vaccinated with pneumococcal vaccine and annually with influenza vaccine. Because cigarette smoking is a risk factor for development of pneumonia, encouraging smoking cessation is another important prevention strategy.[16]

A helpful resource for further details is the CDC's *Guidelines for Preventing Health-Care-Associated Pneumonia, 2003.*[17]

As always, education of healthcare workers is critical. Personnel can transfer healthcare-associated bacteria to patients, yet simple measures such as hand hygiene and use of appropriate barriers and standard precautions with all patients can be very effective prevention. (Guidelines for proper hand hygiene are published by the CDC and the World Health Organization.) Staff members need to have real-time, local data on VAPs fed back to them. Clinicians caring for patients on ventilators should also be educated about use of noninvasive strategies. Surveillance should include "outcomes" such as VAP rates (number of VAP cases divided by number of ventilator days times 1,000) as well as "process" measures including hand hygiene, bed position, daily interruption of sedation and assessment of weaning readiness, and regular oral care. Implement policies and procedures on disinfection, sterilization, and maintenance of respiratory equipment on evidence-based practice. The CDC's *Guidelines for Preventing Healthcare Associated Pneumonia 2003* provides specific information. Lastly, everyone is responsible for the prevention of infection from the CEO to the bedside staff.

Special approaches, according to the SHEA/IDSA *Compendium* report, for use when data and/or risk assessment suggests lack of effective control despite use of basic practices, include:

- Perform a VAP risk assessment

- Use an ET tube with in-line and subglottic suctioning for all eligible patients

- Ensure that all ICU beds for patients undergoing ventilation have a built-in tool to continuously monitor incline angle

BLOODSTREAM INFECTIONS

Almost 40% of all healthcare-associated bacteria infections are due to vascular access in some form and are mostly preventable. The device posing the greatest risk of intravascular device-related bloodstream infection (BSI) is the central venous catheter.[18]

Organisms enter the bloodstream in the following three ways:

- During insertion or days afterward, organisms enter the percutaneous tract

- When the catheter is inserted over a guidewire or later manipulated, organisms contaminate the hub and lumen

- Organisms are carried through the bloodstream to the implanted device from remote sources of infection such as pneumonia[19]

Risk factors[20,21]

Risk factors for central line–associated BSIs (CLABSI) include:

- Prolonged hospitalization before catheterization

- Prolonged catheterization

- Heavy microbial colonization at the insertion site or catheter hub

- Severity of illness

- Underlying neutropenia, AIDS, bone marrow transplant, prematurity

- Extremes of age

- ICU stays

- Femoral vein or jugular vein site versus subclavian site of insertion

- Type of device (with short-term, noncuffed, single or double lumen catheters inserted into subclavian or internal jugular vein having higher rates than surgically implanted cuffed Hickman or Broviac catheters and subclavian central venous ports)

- Total parenteral nutrition

- Substandard care of the catheter (excessive manipulation or a reduced nurse-to-patient ratio)

As with any invasive device, central lines need to be handled with strict asepsis and removed as soon as they are no longer necessary for patient care.

Common etiologic agents

Many cases of central line–associated bacteremia are due to skin organisms such as coagulase-negative *Staphylococcus*, *Staphylococcus aureus*, enteric gram-negative rods, *Pseudomonas aeruginosa*, *Candida*, *Corynebacterium*, and *Enterococcus*.[22]

Prevention and control of CLABSIs

Studies have shown that insertion and maintenance of a catheter by inexperienced staff members might increase the risk of CLABSIs. Education of all healthcare workers and physicians involved in central line insertion, care, and maintenance is key to prevention of these infections.[23] This should occur on hire and must be repeated at least annually. A good way to ensure competence includes having staff members demonstrate procedures. Catheter inserters should undergo credentialing per their organizations to ensure competency before inserting a central vein catheter (CVC). Staff members should complete an education program regarding basic practices to prevent CLABSIs and have periodic reassessments of their knowledge and adherence to these measures. Many facilities make this a fun and engaging activity for the staff by including this in infection prevention or patient safety fairs.

Staffing also affects the occurrence of CLABSIs. Since many of these lines are in patients in ICUs, staffing levels in those units should be addressed.[24]

Rates of infection of CLABSIs per 1,000 days of central lines need to be monitored for trends and reported back to the staff and leadership. If rates are high in one area, this is the time to review practice and, for example, determine whether a catheter insertion checklist and a central line cart or kit containing all items necessary for insertion was used. These are two practical tools to assist the staff in following evidence-based practice. See The Joint Commission's National Patient Safety Goals on prevention of CLABSIs.

Insertion of catheter[25,26]

Most device-related BSIs with a short-term device in place less than 10 days (such as a non-cuffed, non-tunneled CVC) are from skin organisms at the insertion site. However, when a long-term device is in place greater than 10 days (such as cuffed Hickman and Broviac catheters, subcutaneous ports, and peripherally inserted central venous catheter), contamination of the catheter hub and luminal fluid is the major cause of BSIs. Contaminated infusate, while rare, can also cause BSIs.[27]

In adults, avoid the use of the femoral vein, as this site is associated with greater risk of infection and deep venous thrombosis (the jugular site is preferred for hemodialysis access). Of course, it is imperative to use hand hygiene before insertion or manipulation of any IV device, especially central lines, as these lines carry a substantially greater risk of infection than peripheral IVs.

Therefore, use maximal sterile barriers (e.g., a mask, cap, sterile gown, large sterile drape, and sterile gloves), which studies have shown reduce the risk of infection with these lines. These guidelines should also be followed when exchanging a catheter over a guidewire. Insertion of the central line should be observed by a trained healthcare professional to ensure that aseptic technique is followed, and the healthcare professional, using an insertion checklist, should be empowered to stop the procedure if breaches in technique are observed.

Skin flora density at the insertion site is a major risk factor for CLABSIs. Chlorhexidine gluconate (CHG) 2% is the preferred skin antiseptic for line insertion in patients older than two months. Tincture of iodine, an iodophor, or 70% alcohol are also acceptable skin preps.[28]

Sutureless devices should be used to secure the access.

Maintenance of catheter[29,30]

Either sterile gauze or a semipermeable polyurethane dressing should be used for the central line dressing. The dressing should be changed every two days (using gauze) or seven days (using transparent dressing) and also when damp, loose, or soiled.

Antimicrobial ointments are not routinely recommended for central line insertion, with the exception of povidone-iodine or polysporin ointment at hemodialysis catheter insertion sites in patients with a recurrent history of *Staphylococcus aureus* CLABSIs.

Before accessing the catheter, disinfect the hub, needleless connectors, and injection ports with alcoholic CHG prep, or 70% alcohol. Then, monitor the site daily. Assess the need for the catheter daily during multidisciplinary rounds, and remove it as soon as it is no longer required for patient care.

All administration sets (except those used for blood, blood products, or lipids) should be replaced no more frequently than every 96 hours, including caps and needleless connectors. Do not routinely replace central venous catheters, such as peripherally inserted central catheters or arterial catheters, solely for the purposes of reducing the incidence of infection or in patients whose only indication of infection is fever. Such replacements should only take place when catheter infection is suspected. The catheter should also be replaced if purulent, as noted at the exit site, especially if the patient is hemodynamically unstable or a CLABSI is suspected.

For adults, if the facility rate of CLABSI is high despite the use of the previously mentioned measures and the catheter is likely to remain in place for more than five days, use an antimicrobial-coated or antiseptic-impregnated central venous catheter.

Per the *Compendium of Strategies,* special approaches should be used when unacceptably high CLABSI rates occur despite implementation of the basic CLABSI prevention strategies listed earlier in this chapter. These include:

- Bathe ICU patients older than 2 months of age with a chlorhexidine gluconate preparation on a daily basis

- Use a povidone-iodine preparation to clean CVC insertion sites for children younger than 2 months of age, especially low-birth-weight neonates

- Use antiseptic- or antimicrobial-impregnated CVCs for adult patients

- Use CHG-containing sponge dressings for CVCs in patients older than 2 months of age

- Use antimicrobial locks for CVCs in very select situations (see *The Compendium* for examples)

SURGICAL SITE INFECTIONS

SSIs occur in 2% to 5% of patients undergoing inpatient surgery in the Unites States.[31] They make up the third most frequent HAI among hospital patients, increasing the likelihood of ICU stays by 60%.[32] The source of most SSIs is the patient's own endogenous flora.

The risk of infection is determined by the following four factors:

- Wound contamination or bacterial inoculum

- The virulence of the organisms

- The microenvironment of the wound

- The local and systemic defenses of the host[33]

SSI risk is related to the number of organisms contaminating the wound. A decreased number of organisms is required for infection if there is a foreign body present. Some organisms are more virulent or disease-producing, such as Group A *Streptococcus,* which requires only a small number of organisms to cause severe infection. The local environment of the surgical wound can be predisposed to infection, such as hematomas, necrotic tissue, or the presence of foreign material. Local host defenses also play a role in the risk of SSI. Factors such as morbid obesity, remote infection at other sites, cancer, diabetes, and immunosuppressive therapy can increase the risk of infection at the surgical site.

Each SSI is associated with approximately seven to 10 additional postoperative hospital days. Patients who develop an SSI have a two to 11 times higher risk of death, compared with the operative patient without an SSI. Attributable costs vary with estimates from $3,000 to $29,000.[34]

Risk factors

A variety of factors may influence the risk of SSIs. Although age is not modifiable, other risk factors may be, such as glucose control in diabetics, obesity, nutrition, and cessation of smoking within 30 days before surgery. In the perioperative period, immunosuppressive medications should be avoided if possible.

The length of the preoperative stay has been noted at times as a risk factor for SSI; however, it may be more of an indication of comorbid conditions in patients that require longer stays.

Preoperative risk factors include the method of hair removal as well as presence of remote infection. During the operative period, factors such as surgical team members' scrub, patient skin prep, and antimicrobial prophylaxis (choice, timing, and duration) can affect the patient's risk of infection in addition to operation time, asepsis, and surgical skill. In terms of the operating room itself, the ventilation, traffic, environmental surfaces, and, of course, proper sterilization of instruments are all risk factors.

Controlling blood glucose during the immediate postoperative period for patients undergoing cardiac surgery has also been shown to affect infection rates.

Surveillance for SSI rates, process measures, and feedback to surgeons, perioperative staff members, and leadership can significantly affect SSI rates. Staff members must know there is a problem to be able to change their practice for improved outcomes.

Common etiologic agents

Staphylococcus aureus, coagulase-negative *staphylococci, Enterococcus spp.,* and *E. coli* are frequently isolated pathogens. An increasing proportion of SSIs are caused by antimicrobial-resistant pathogens, such as methicillin-resistant *Staphylococcus aureus* or other organisms such as *Candida albicans.*[35]

Prevention[36]

CDC surgical site guidelines state that hair should not be removed unless it will interfere with the surgery. If removal is necessary, clippers should be used. The increased infection risk associated with shaving is related to the fact that microscopic nicks in the skin may provide a portal of entry for microorganisms to multiply. To lower infection rates, clipping should be done immediately before surgery versus the night before.

Preoperative infection remote to the surgical site, such as UTIs, should be treated prior to elective surgery so as not to seed the operative site; alternatively, surgery should be postponed until the infection has cleared.

Scrub team members should perform a two- to six-minute preoperative surgical scrub with an appropriate antiseptic agent with persistent action, or use an alcohol-based surgical hand antisepsis product. The hands and forearms, up to the elbows, should be scrubbed.

It is important to note that a team member who wears artificial nails may have hand colonization with bacteria and fungi despite an adequate scrub. Team members should not wear artificial nails or extenders and should keep natural nails less than one-quarter of an inch long.[37]

Instruct patients to shower or bathe with an antiseptic agent on at least the night before surgery. Thoroughly wash and clean at and around the incision site to remove gross contamination before application of the skin preparation. Use an appropriate antiseptic agent for skin preparation. Apply the skin preparation in concentric circles, moving toward the periphery to make the prepared area large enough to extend the incision or create new incisions or drain sites, if necessary.

Surgical prophylaxis refers to a very brief course of an antimicrobial initiated just before an operation begins, critically timed, to reduce the burden of intraoperative contamination to a level that won't overwhelm the host defenses. Several groups, including the Surgical Infection Prevention Collaborative and Surgical Care Improvement Project through Centers for Medicare & Medicaid Services, as well as the CDC, address surgical antimicrobial prophylaxis. It is recommended to administer a prophylactic antimicrobial only when indicated and based on the surgical procedure, the most common pathogen causing SSI for a specific procedure, and published recommendations. The key with prophylaxis is not only the choice of agent but timing and duration of therapy. The drug should be administered within one hour before incision to maximize the concentration in the tissues. Prophylaxis should also be discontinued within 24 hours after all procedures except cardiac surgery, for which it should be stopped within 48 hours. Many hospitals that have followed these measures have decreased their SSI rates.

The surgeon as well as the professional nurse in the operating room set the tone for surgery. Aseptic technique should be strictly followed whether starting an intravascular line, inserting an epidural catheter for anesthesia, administering sterile medications, or performing surgery on the patient. Standard principles of asepsis in the operating room should be followed. Sterile equipment and solutions should be assembled immediately prior to surgery and not opened and prepared ahead of time or covered up with a sterile drape. The surgeon and staff should handle tissue gently while maintaining effective hemostasis and eradicating dead space. Operative time should be minimized as much as possible.

The operating room should be under positive pressure with respect to adjacent corridors and maintain ventilation of at least 15 air exchanges per hour, with three of these being fresh air. All air should be filtered appropriately per the American Institute of Architects' recommendations, introduced at the ceiling, and exhausted at the floor. Only necessary personnel should enter the operating room, and its door should remain closed at all times, except to allow entrance and egress to people, equipment, and the patient.

Operating room surfaces and equipment should be cleaned with an Environmental Protection Agency–approved hospital disinfectant. *AORN Standards, Recommended Practices, and Guidelines* for environmental cleaning should be followed. The Association of periOperative Registered Nurses (AORN) recommends the "contain and confine" principle in terms of contamination. It also recommends that operating rooms be cleaned before and after each surgical procedure and at the end of the day (terminal cleaning). Terminally cleaning all surgical procedure rooms and scrub/utility areas regardless of whether they are used is recommended. Terminal cleaning also involves not only all horizontal surfaces, but also every item in the rooms, such as surgical lights and tracks, fixed and ceiling-mounted equipment, all furniture including wheels and casters, hallways and floors, cabinet handles and push plates, ventilation faceplates, substerile areas, scrub/utility areas, and scrub sinks.

Proper cleaning and sterilization of instruments according to published guidelines, such as those from the CDC and AORN, is crucial in the prevention of infection at the surgical site. Sterilization should be used only for instruments that will be used immediately and should not be used for convenience or as an alternative to purchasing additional inventory.

The *Compendium*[38] notes that blood glucose should be controlled during the immediate postoperative period for patients undergoing heart surgery. Blood glucose levels should be maintained at less than 200 mg/dL. The blood glucose level should be measured at 6 a.m. on postoperative days one and two, with the procedure date being postoperative day zero. This *Compendium of Strategies* notes that initiating blood glucose control in the intraoperative period has not been shown to reduce the risk of SSI as compared to postoperatively and may actually lead to higher rates of adverse outcomes.

The Joint Commission's National Patient Safety Goals include implementing best practices to prevent SSIs. Many of these issues are addressed in these standards, along with periodic risk assessments for SSIs and monitoring of compliance with best practices. Education plays a major role in prevention of infection at the surgical site. The facility should educate healthcare workers involved in surgical procedures upon hiring, annually, and when involvement in the procedures is added to an individual's job responsibilities. The facility should also educate patients who will undergo surgery, and their families, as needed, regarding prevention of SSI.

Finally, the surgical team needs to be aware of SSI rates. Feedback should be provided to team leaders, individual surgeons, hospital leadership, and perioperative staff members. Data should be provided confidentially to individual surgeons, the department, and/or department chiefs. The surgical team also needs to know how well it is complying with process measures, such as the percentage of procedures in which antimicrobial prophylaxis was appropriately provided (administration of correct agent, within one hour before incision [two hours are allowed for vancomycin and fluoroquinolones], and stopping agent within 24 hours after surgery [48 hours for heart surgery]). Other process measures suggested for monitoring are compliance with hair removal guidelines and compliance with perioperative glucose control guidelines, among others.

Special approaches[39]

Special approaches should be used, per the *Compendium of Strategies,* when unacceptably high SSI rates are occurring despite implementation of the basic SSI prevention strategies listed previously. These include:

- Perform expanded SSI surveillance to determine the source and extent of the problem and to identify possible targets for intervention
- Expand surveillance (aligned with the hospital's strategic plan) to include additional procedures and possibly to all National Healthcare Safety Network procedures

CONCLUSION

UTIs, pneumonias, bloodstream infections, and SSIs comprise the majority of HAIs detected in patients in many settings. Infection preventionists must be familiar with risk factors for these infections as well as preventive measures specific for each site of infection. Our patient outcomes are at stake.

REFERENCES

1. D. Leithauser, "Urinary Tract Infections," *APIC Text Infection Control and Epidemiology 2005*, Second Edition (Washington, DC: APIC, 2005).

2. Ibid.

3. Carolyn V. Gould, et al., *Draft Guidelines For Prevention of Catheter-Associated Urinary Tract Infections, 2009* (CDC, 2009).

4. Ibid.

5. E. Lo, et al., "Strategies to Prevent Catheter-Associated Urinary Tract Infections in Acute Care Hospitals: A Compendium of Strategies to Prevent Healthcare-Associated Infections in Acute Care Hospitals," *Infection Control and Hospital Epidemiology* 29.1 (2008): S41–S50.

6. Ibid.

7. Carolyn V. Gould, et al.

8. Edward S. Wong, Thomas M. Hooton, *CDC Guideline for Prevention of Catheter-Associated Urinary Tract Infections* (CDC, 1981).

9. *Guide to the Elimination of Catheter-Associated Urinary Tract Infection: Developing and Applying Facility-Based Prevention Interventions in Acute and Long-Term Care Settings* (Washington, DC: APIC, 2008).

10. Ibid.

11. D. Christensen, "Pneumonia," *APIC Text of Infection Control and Epidemiology, 2005, Second Edition,* (Washington, DC: APIC, 2005).

12. L. R. Greene, et. al., *APIC Elimination Guide: Guide to the Elimination of Ventilator-Associated Pneumonia, 2009* (Washington, DC: APIC, 2009).

13. D. Christensen.

14. S.E. Coffin, et al., "Strategies to Prevent Ventilator-Associated Pneumonia in Acute Care Hospitals," *Infection Control and Hospital Epidemiology* 29.1 (2008): S31–S40.

15. D. Christensen

16. O.C. Tablan, et al., "Guidelines for Preventing Health-Care-Associated Pneumonia, 2003: Recommendations of CDC and the Healthcare Infection Control Practices Advisory Committee," *Morbidity and Mortality Weekly Report* RR-3 (2003).

17. Ibid.

18. C.J. Crnich, D.G. Maki., "Intravascular Device Infections," APIC *Text of Infection Control and Epidemiology 2005*, Second Edition (Washington DC: APIC, 2005).

19. Ibid.

20. Ibid.

21. J. Marshall, et al., "Strategies to Prevent Central Line-Associated Infections in Acute Care Hospitals in Acute Care Hospitals: A Compendium of Strategies to Prevent Healthcare-Associated Infections in Acute Care Hospitals," *Infections Control and Hospital Epidemiology* 29.1 (2008): S22–S30.

22. C.J. Crnich, D.G. Maki.

23. J. Marshall, et al.

24. N.P. O'Grady, et al., "Guidelines for Hand Hygiene in Healthcare Settings: Recommendations of the Healthcare Infection Control Practices Advisory Committee," *Morbidity and Mortality Weekly Report* RR-10 (2002): 1–26.

25. J. Marshall, et al.

26. N.P. O'Grady, et al.

27. C.J. Crnich, D.G. Maki.

28. N.P. O'Grady, et al., "Guidelines for the Prevention of Intravascular Catheter-Related Infections," *Morbidity and Mortality Weekly Report,* RR-10 (2002): 1–26.

29. Ibid.

30. J. Marshall, et al.

31. Deverick J. Anderson, et al., "Strategies to Prevent Surgical Site Infections in Acute Care Hospitals: A Compendium of Strategies to Prevent Healthcare-Associated Infections in Acute Care Hospitals," *Infection Control and Hospital Epidemiology 2008* 29.1 (2008): S51–S61.

32. J. Janelle, et al., "Surgical Site Infections," APIC *Text of Infection Control and Epidemiology 2005, Second Edition* (Washington, DC: APIC, 2005).

33. Ibid.

34. Deverick J. Anderson, et al.

35. A.J. Mangram, et al., "HICPAC Guidelines for the Prevention of Surgical Site Infections, 1999," *Infection Control and Hospital Epidemiology* 4 (1999): 247–278.

36. Ibid.

37. J.M. Boyce, D. Pittet, "CDC Guidelines for Hand Hygiene in Healthcare Settings: Recommendations of the Healthcare Infection Control Practices Advisory Committee and the HICPAC/SHEA/APIC/IDSA Hand Hygiene Task Force," *Morbidity and Mortality Weekly Report* RR-16 (2002): 1–45.

38. Deverick J. Anderson, et al.

39. Ibid.

Antimicrobial-Resistant Organisms

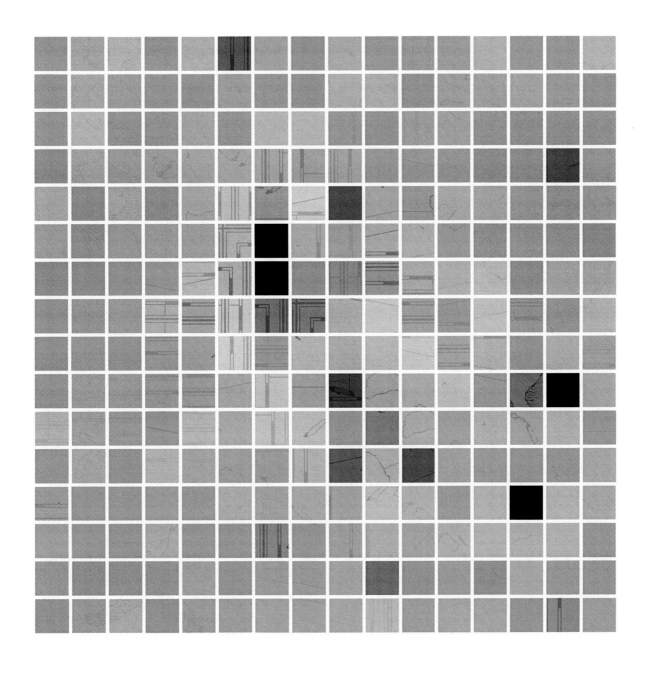

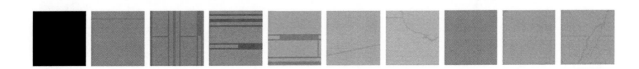

Antimicrobial-Resistant Organisms

According to the Centers for Disease Control and Prevention (CDC), "the prevention and control of multidrug-resistant organisms (MDRO) is a national priority—one that requires that all healthcare facilities and agencies assume responsibility."[1] No healthcare setting has escaped the effect of these resistant microbes. The CDC states that "more than 70% of the bacteria that cause hospital-associated infections are resistant to at least one of the drugs used to treat them."[2] Such resistance is why it is important that an infection preventionist (IP) pays attention to and collects data on MDROs.

MDROs are bacteria and other organisms that have developed resistance to one or more classes of antimicrobial drugs. Options for treatment are often very limited. Common examples of these organisms include:

- Methicillin (or oxacillin)-resistant *Staphylococcus aureus* (MRSA)

- Vancomycin-resistant enterococci (VRE)

- Vancomycin-intermediate *Staphylococcus aureus* (VISA)

- Vancomycin-resistant *Staphylococcus aureus* (VRSA)

- Extended-spectrum beta-lactamases (ESBL), which are resistant to cephalosporins and monobactams

- Carbapenemase-resistant *Enterobacter* (CRE)

- Others

Patients may be colonized or infected with these organisms. **Colonization** is the presence of the organism in or on the body without any symptoms, such as MRSA found in a culture of the nares.

Infection occurs when the organism multiplies and invades the tissues and causes symptoms and illness.

Risk factors for MDROs include:

- Severity of illness

- Previous antimicrobial exposure

- Underlying illness such as chronic renal disease, diabetes mellitus, peripheral vascular disease, and dermatitis or skin lesions

- Repeated healthcare system contact

- Colonization by an MDRO

- Invasive devices

- Advanced age

Person-to-person transmission by the hands of healthcare workers (direct contact) appears to be the most common mode of spread. Therefore, strategies to monitor adherence to hand hygiene and glove use are critical. MDROs add considerably to increased length of stay (due to morbidity), mortality, and cost for patients and residents, especially in the acute and long-term care settings where patients shuttle back and forth between settings. During the past several decades, MDROs have increased steadily in hospitals and medical centers.

Transmission of resistant strains are influenced by:

- Numbers of available vulnerable patients

- Antimicrobial pressure

- Increased potential for spread from large numbers of colonized or infected patients

- Adherence to known prevention measures

MRSA

"MRSA is the most common pathogen causing [healthcare-acquired infections] in healthcare facilities in the United States and throughout the world. Today, MRSA accounts for as many as 50%–70% of the *S[taphylococcus] aureus* infections acquired in healthcare facilities (and *S[taphylococcus] aureus* is the most common hospital pathogen)."[3] MRSA has also spread to the community as community-acquired MRSA and usually causes skin and soft tissue infections, whereas healthcare-associated MRSA usually causes bloodstream, surgical site, pneumonia, or urinary tract infections.

According to the *APIC National Prevalence Study on MRSA,* 46 out of every 1,000 patients in the study were either infected or colonized with MRSA (21% of all U.S. healthcare facilities participated in the study). Seventy-seven percent were detected within less than 48 hours of admission, and 23% were detected within more than 48 hours of admission. This rate is eight to 11 times greater than previous MRSA estimates.[4]

Risk factors

Risk factors for MRSA include:

- Hospital admission in the previous year with at least one underlying chronic illness
- Admission to a nursing home in the previous year
- Prior receipt of antibiotics during an admission
- Skin and soft tissue infection at admission
- HIV infection
- Injection drug use
- Previous infection or colonization with MRSA
- Hemodialysis
- Risk factors specific to your facility[5]

Transmission

Direct skin-to-skin contact (hands of healthcare workers) as well as indirect contact (contact with contaminated surfaces and environment) are responsible for transmission of MRSA. Therefore, hand hygiene and cleaning of equipment and the patient's environment are crucial in interrupting transmission of this organism.

Prevention and control

The following is a summary of components that the Association for Professionals in Infection Control and Epidemiology (APIC) recommends facilities have in place to prevent transmission of MRSA:

- **MRSA risk assessment.** By using past and current MRSA surveillance data, the IP can develop a plan for MRSA surveillance, prevention, and control specific to the facility's unique risks.

- **MRSA surveillance program.** Based on the risk assessment, the surveillance program outlines a plan for goals, interventions to reach those goals, and evaluation of the interventions. Consistent communication with the microbiology laboratory must undergird this effort, and results of the surveillance must be fed back to the staff members/providers.

- **Hand hygiene.** Proper hand hygiene must be monitored and enforced, as this is the main mode of transmission of the organism.

- **Contact precautions.** Recommended by the CDC for acute care especially, contact precautions involve the use of gloves and gown each time a healthcare worker enters the room as well as properly placing the patient, preferably in a private room or cohorting as an alternative; if these are not options, the roommate must be carefully evaluated for risk of acquisition of MRSA and have a shorter length of stay.

- **Environmental and equipment cleaning and disinfection.** MRSA can survive for almost two months in the environment (e.g., on charts, tabletops, and cloth curtains); therefore, proper cleaning is essential to control transmission. Environmental services and nursing staff members must be taught proper cleaning techniques.

- **Targeted active surveillance cultures.** Facilities must decide whether to test only high-risk patients (e.g., long-term care residents, patients with recent or frequent hospitalizations, dialysis patients, athletes, veterinarians, patients with a history of IV drug use or prison stay, or unique high-risk groups to the facility) or all patients admitted to the facility. Facilities should also check state laws for any requirements. Timing is critical, as rapid detection allows for quicker initiation of contact precautions and possible treatment to limit spreading the infection.

- **Decolonization.** Use this strategy only in specific circumstances, such as when elimination of MRSA has been suggested as a control and prevention measure because of ongoing transmission of MRSA in a well-defined cohort having close contact. Also use as a strategy if a physician determines that a patient may benefit clinically from decolonization.

- **Antimicrobial stewardship.** This is an essential strategy to affect sustainable, long-term management of MRSA.

- **Cultural transformation.** When change comes from within your staff members (e.g., from a staff champion or multidisciplinary team solutions), the change is likely to be more accepted and long lasting.

- **Administrative support.** This is crucial to any MRSA-prevention efforts. Sharing success stories from other facilities is urged as well. Any real or perceived barriers to participation in your facility, trends (including incidence and prevalence rates of MRSA), costs to the facility of a healthcare-associated infection (HAI), and any pertinent literature should also be shared. It is important to convince administration that an ounce of prevention is truly worth a pound of cure.[6]

VRE

Enterococci make up part of the normal human gastrointestinal flora and female genital tract (colonization) and are often found in the environment. Sometimes they cause infection, usually of the urinary tract, bloodstream, or a wound. *Enterococcus faecalis* and *Enterococcus faecium* are the most common enterococcal isolates. Vancomycin is often used to treat enterococcal infection, but these organisms have become resistant to vancomycin. This is especially worrisome as there is a potential for vancomycin-resistant genes to transfer to more virulent organisms such as *Staphylococcus aureus*.

Risk factors

According to the CDC, those at risk for VRE infection include people who:

- Have been previously treated with the antibiotic vancomycin or other antibiotics for long periods of time

- Are hospitalized, particularly when they receive antibiotic treatment for long periods of time

- Have weakened immune systems, such as patients in the ICU or in cancer or transplant wards

- Have undergone surgical procedures, such as abdominal or chest surgery

- Have medical devices that stay in for extended lengths of time, such as urinary catheters or central IV catheters

- Are colonized with VRE[7]

According to the CDC, enterococci caused one of eight infections in hospitals in 2006 and 2007, but only about 30% of these were due to VRE.

Transmission

VRE is spread person to person (direct contact) by the hands of healthcare workers and from contact with contaminated items in the environment.

Prevention and control

The Joint Commission recently included prevention of HAIs due to MDROs in acute care in its National Patient Safety Goals. The Joint Commission, like APIC, has stated that a risk assessment needs to be conducted periodically for MDROs to plan your strategies. With VRE, the same prevention and control measures are needed as with MRSA, such as hand hygiene, contact precautions, and strict environmental and equipment cleaning and disinfection, as it can persist on a variety of environmental surfaces. In addition, The Joint Commission calls for a lab-based alert system to identify patients with MDROs and also an alert system that identifies readmitted or transferred MDRO-positive patients. For more guidelines and standards, refer to the CDC's *HICPAC Guidelines on Management of Multi-drug Resistant Organisms in Healthcare Settings, 2006,* which can be found at *www.cdc.gov/ncidod/dhqp/hicpac.html.*

VISA/VRSA

According to the CDC, the first documented case of VISA was reported in Japan in 1996.[8] Treatment of MRSA infections and empirical therapy where MRSA prevalence was high has led to development of VISA (minimum inhibitory concentration [MIC] = 4–8 µg/mL). In this same report, as of 2006, there were six reported VRSA (MIC = $\geq$ 16 µg/mL) infections reported in patients in the United States. This is especially concerning because VISA strains are refractory to treatment with vancomycin, particularly when indwelling catheters are present or there is an unidentified focus of infection; also, vancomycin is ineffective for treatment of VRSA infections. Again, the same basic infection control measures apply as for all MDROs with strict use of hand hygiene, a private room, contact precautions, dedication of nondisposable equipment that cannot be cleaned and disinfected between patients, and minimization of the number of persons caring for the patient (i.e., dedicated staff members). These precautions may need to be customized to other special settings. A contact investigation may be warranted on a case-by-case basis according to the CDC.[9]

ESBL ENTEROBACTERIACAE

Increased use of beta-lactam antibiotics (i.e., penicillins, cephalosporins, carbapenems, and mono-bactams), especially third-generation cephalosporins, have been associated with the emergence of beta-lactamases—enzymes that cause resistance and lead to extended spectrum beta-lactamase–producing bacteria. Some organisms that produce ESBLs include *Klebsiella pneumonia, Klebsiella oxytoca, E. coli, Salmonella spp., Proteus mirabilis,* and *Pseudomonas aeruginosa.* These organisms are difficult to treat because they carry plasmids that confer resistance to many antibiotics.

Risk factors

Patients at high risk for ESBLs include:

- Neutropenic patients

- Transplant recipients

- Premature neonates

- Elderly persons

- Patients with prolonged/extensive antibiotic use (e.g., cephalosporins)

- Post-gastrointestinal surgery patients

High-risk units include:

- ICUs

- Hematology/oncology units

- Transplant units

- Long-term/chronic care facilities[10]

Transmission

Patient-to-patient spread of the infection through the contaminated hands of healthcare workers is thought to be the major means of transmission, although some outbreaks have involved contaminated medical devices (e.g., ultrasound gel).

Prevention and control

According to the reference above, five common theme interventions comprise best practices:

- Antibiotic stewardship

- Surveillance and screening

- Contact precautions

- Hand hygiene

- Disinfection (environment and equipment)

Let's discuss surveillance screening specifically. The microbiology lab must be enlisted to report and isolate, and then the IP must assess patient risk factors and place the patient on contact precautions. A risk assessment should be performed by calculating incidence and prevalence of infection/colonization of ESBLs. Once ESBLs are endemic or prevalent in your facility or area, you need to consider the possibility of screening high-risk populations or all admissions to high-risk units as noted earlier.

The perianal/rectal area and urine are most commonly cultured because the organisms are usually found there. Rescreening during the admission can occur if ESBL-associated risk factors change.

With the use of contact precautions, ensure a private room or cohort patients with similar conditions. If you must place a patient with ESBL with a non-ESBL patient, make sure that the non-ESBL patient does not have risk factors such as indwelling devices, a transplant history, or neutropenia. Meticulous cleaning, especially of frequently touched surfaces and patient care equipment, should occur.

CARBAPENEMASE-RESISTANT *ENTEROBACTER*

In *Morbidity and Mortality Weekly Report,* the CDC issued guidance for control of CRE or carbapenemase-producing *Enterobacteriacae* as an emerging pathogen.[11] Currently, carbapenem-resistant *Klebsiella pneumonia* (CRKP) is the most common species of CRE in the United States and is resistant to almost all of the available antimicrobials, according to the CDC. Association has occurred between CRKP infection and high rates of morbidity and mortality, especially in patients with prolonged hospitalization, those who are critically ill, and those exposed to invasive devices. In addition to having been isolated in 24 states thus far, it is now found routinely in some hospitals in New York and New Jersey. This is another worrisome issue concerning antimicrobial resistance to Gram-negative bacteria and calls for aggressive detection to control the organism now before it becomes more endemic throughout the country.

Risk factors

Risk factors are the same as many other drug-resistant organisms:

- Very long preinfection stays in hospitals (e.g., 25 days compared to six days)

- Underlying diseases

- Invasive devices (e.g., central lines and ventilators)

- Exposure to ICUs

- Prior exposure to antibiotics, especially carbapenems

Transmission, prevention and control

Transmission of CREs appears to be direct and indirect contact, as with many MDROs. The following are prevention and control tips adapted from the CDC:[12]

- All acute care facilities should use contact precautions for infected/colonized patients with these organisms. No recommendation can be made for how long to use the precautions. Hand hygiene should be strictly enforced.

- Because some strains of *Enterobacteriacae* have elevated MICs but are still within the "susceptible" range of carbapenems, they would not be identified as potential clinical or infection control risks. Therefore, clinical labs should follow Clinical and Laboratory Standards Institute guidelines for susceptibility testing and establish a protocol for detection of carbapenemase production (e.g., the modified Hodge test).

- Any *Enterobacteriacae* isolate that is nonsusceptible to carbapenems or *Klebsiella spp.* or *E. coli* isolates that test positive for carbepenemase should be reported promptly to the infection prevention staff.

- All acute care facilities should review culture results for the preceding six to 12 months to determine whether previously unrecognized CRE has been present in their facility. If CRE is identified, then a single round of active surveillance cultures (i.e., a point-prevalence survey) should be done in high-risk units (e.g., ICUs, units where cases have been identified, units where many patients are exposed to broad spectrum antimicrobials) to look for CRE.

- Surveillance specimens might include stool specimens, rectal swabs, or perirectal swabs.

- If no previous unrecognized CRE is identified, then monitoring for clinical infection should be continued.

- If CRE or carbapenemase-producing *Klebsiella ssp.* or *E. coli* are detected in one or more cultures, or if unrecognized colonization is found, the facility should investigate by conducting active surveillance of patients with epidemiological links to patients with CRE infection (patients in the same unit or who have been cared for by the same healthcare personnel).

- Continued active surveillance weekly until no new cases of colonization or infection are detected.

- If transmission of CRE is not identified after repeated active surveillance testing, consider performing periodic point-prevalence surveys in high-risk units. In areas where CRE is endemic, an increased likelihood of CRE importation exists; therefore, monitor clinical cases and consider additional strategies as described in the *2006 Tier 2 CDC Guidelines for Management of Multidrug-Resistant Organisms in Healthcare Settings.*[13]

OTHER MDROS

There are other MDROs of significance, but we will only cover *Acinetobacter* and *Clostridium difficile (C. diff)*.

Acinetobacter

Acinetobacter are nonfermenting Gram-negative coccobacilli commonly found in soil and water and on skin of healthy persons about 25% of the time,[14] especially on the skin of healthcare workers. These organisms can also survive on dry surfaces for long periods and can most likely be transmitted via dust and fomites.[15] Although there are numerous types of *Acinetobacter*, *Acinetobacter baumannii,* formerly known as *Acinetobacter calcoacetus var. anitratus,* causes 80% of infections.[16] *Acinetobacter baumannii* has even been dubbed "Iraqibacter" by U.S. troops, as it is prevalent in up to 20% of the wounded returning home from Iraq and Afghanistan.[17] Many clinical isolates of *Acinetobacter* represent colonization, but outbreaks of *Acinetobacter* usually occur in very ill patients in ICUs. *Acinetobacter* is an uncommon pathogen, and infections rarely occur outside of healthcare settings or in healthy people. *Acinetobacter* may cause bacteremia, pneumonia, meningitis, urinary infections, and endocarditis. Multidrug resistance has been reported as well as outbreaks. Some long-term care facilities are admitting patients who are colonized or infected with this organism.

Risk factors

Risk factors for *Acinetobacter* include:

- Weakened immune systems, such as in the immunocompromised or debilitated hosts
- Chronic lung disease
- Diabetes
- Very ill hospitalized patients
- Ventilator patients
- Open wounds
- Prolonged hospital stay
- Prior broad-spectrum antibiotic therapy[18]

Transmission

Acinetobacter are transmitted by person-to-person contact, contact with contaminated surfaces, or exposure in the environment.

Prevention and control

The routine basics of infection control apply to all MDROs, including hand hygiene, use of contact precautions by some facilities (especially if the organism is very resistant, or only susceptible to one or two classes of antibiotics), and strict environmental cleaning and disinfection. Also, notification of other areas of the facility or other facilities should occur when a patient with *Acinetobacter* is transferred.

Clostridium difficile

C. diff, although not really considered an MDRO, is an organism of epidemiologic significance, and for this reason, is discussed in this chapter. *C. diff* is a spore-forming, anaerobic Gram-positive bacillus found in the intestines. One study states that "it has been estimated that 3% of healthy adults and 20%–40% of hospitalized patients are colonized with *C. diff* but are asymptomatic until exposure to antibiotics."[19] *C. diff* is now competing with MRSA in terms of being the most common organism to cause HAIs in the United States.[20]

Many patients with *C. diff* infection may have acquired the pathogen during previous healthcare facility admissions. This organism secretes two toxins (A and B) that cause inflammation of the bowel and profound diarrhea by attacking the epithelial lining of the bowel. There are many strains of *C. diff* (some non-toxigenic), but a newly identified strain, BI/NAP1/027, is so virulent that it produces 16–23 times greater amounts of toxin.[21]

C. diff infection ranges from asymptomatic colonization, diarrhea, pseudomembranous colitis, toxic megacolon, sepsis, and death.

Risk factors

Exposure to antibiotics is the most common risk factor. Nearly all antimicrobials have been implicated in *C. diff* infection, but cephalosporins, clindamycin, and fluoroquinolones seem to cause a high risk for infection.[22] Other risk factors include:

- Gastrointestinal procedures and surgery
- Advanced age

- Indiscriminate use of antibiotics

- Hospitalization or a stay in a nursing home

However, of interest are some severe cases among healthy peripartum women, children, and other healthy people in the community with no recent healthcare contact or antimicrobial exposure.[23]

Dale Gerding notes in the *APIC Text of Infection Control and Epidemiology* that "it was previously believed that the responsible organism, *C. difficile*, is part of the normal flora and proliferates to cause disease when antibiotics are given."[24] Several studies suggest this in incorrect. Patients who are asymptomatically colonized with *C. diff* are actually at decreased risk of disease compared to patients in the same hospital environment not previously colonized with the organism. Patients may be colonized from contact with the contaminated environment or contaminated healthcare workers' hands. But for disease to occur, it is generally accepted that the patient must have received antimicrobials that disrupt the normal flora.

Transmission

Signs and symptoms of *C. diff* include watery diarrhea, three or more bowel movements per day for two or more days (some studies report up to 20 bowel movements per day), fever, loss of appetite, nausea, and abdominal cramping or tenderness. Transmission occurs most commonly from contaminated healthcare workers' hands, medical equipment, or the environment. Patients with *C. diff* should be placed on contact precautions. Spores remain active for months in the environment in soil, on dry surfaces, and especially in places where fecal contamination may occur (e.g., rectal thermometers, bedside commodes, and high-touch surfaces in patient bathrooms such as light switches).

APIC's *Guide to the Elimination of* Clostridium difficile *in Healthcare Settings* notes that transmission can occur in the following activities:

- Sharing rectal electronic thermometers

- Oral care/oral suctioning when hands and items are contaminated

- Administering feedings or medications with contaminated hands, foods, or medications

- Emergency procedures (intubation)

- Poor hand hygiene (proper hygiene is needed even during brief encounters)

- Inconsistent disinfection of equipment

- Sharing patient care items without appropriate disinfection

- Ineffective environmental cleaning

Of note, ongoing transmission may be a marker for poor adherence to environmental decontamination, hand hygiene compliance, and other prevention measures.

Prevention and control

Only watery or loose stools should be tested for C. *diff.* Sometimes, merely stopping the offending antibiotic, if possible, may stop the diarrhea. At other times, oral metronidazole or oral vancomycin may be needed for treatment.

A bundle of interventions has been proposed for management of C. *diff.*[25] All the interventions in the bundle should be implemented for prevention and control. These include:

- Risk assessment for C. *diff*

- Surveillance system for those with diarrhea on admission or who develop diarrhea after admission (i.e., early recognition and an alert system)

- Contact precautions (e.g., hand hygiene and wearing gloves and gown) for patients with diarrhea until test results are returned

- Enforcement of hand washing with soap and water to remove the spores

- Use of an Environmental Protection Agency–approved germicide for routine disinfection (non-outbreaks) and bleach for environmental disinfection in C. *diff* rooms (routine and terminal cleaning) in an outbreak

- Monitoring of hand hygiene, contact precautions, and cleaning and disinfection

- Antimicrobial stewardship

Practical tips

Designate a bedpan/bedside commode solely for the use of the C. *diff* resident, especially in semiprivate rooms. However, it may be more beneficial to let the C. *diff* patient use the bathroom, if able, and have a bedside commode available for the noninfected roommate. This allows for less frequent handling of the C. *diff*–contaminated items.

Develop intake and output sheets with space to mark the number of liquid stool; if the patient is taking an antibiotic and a number other than zero is entered, this may trigger the physician to consider C. *diff* testing.

Also, make sure that cleaning supplies are kept with portable equipment such as blood pressure equipment, portable x-ray machines, etc.[26] Consider whether wipes are big enough. Multiple wipes may be needed to decontaminate an item.

Remember, bleach is corrosive and should not be used on all surfaces. It can be purchased pre-mixed with detergent or mixed fresh daily; don't mix with other chemicals.

Dirty equipment and a dirty environment are major risk factors, so determine who is responsible for cleaning and disinfecting each piece of patient care equipment and all areas of the environment. Don't forget such items as call bells, remote controls, phones, oxygen concentrators, IV pumps, shower chairs, wheelchairs, walkers, bed rails, handrails, and bedside tables.

CONCLUSION

Successful control of MDROs has occurred through a variety of combined strategies, which include, according to the *American Journal of Infection Control* "hand hygiene, use of contact precautions until patients are culture-negative for a target MDRO, active surveillance cultures, education-enhanced environmental cleaning, and improvements in communication about patients with MDROs within and between healthcare facilities."[27] *The American Journal of Infection Control* also states that "nearly all studies reporting successful MDRO control employed a median of seven to eight interventions concurrently or sequentially.[28]

The IP must work to develop a comprehensive, unrelenting program for controlling MDROs, conduct frequent reassessments, and create a tiered strategy of more stringent interventions over time if needed. CDC guidelines have excellent information to guide the IP in this area.

REFERENCES

1. J.D. Siegel, E. Rhinehart, M. Jackson, L. Chiarello, "Management of Multidrug-Resistant Organisms in Healthcare Settings," The Healthcare Practices Infection Control Advisory Committee, CDC, *www.cdc.gov/ncidod/dhqp/pdf/ar/mdroguideline2006.pdf* (2006).

2. "Campaign to Prevent Antimicrobial Resistance in Healthcare Settings," CDC, *www.cdc.gov/drugresistance/healthcare/problem.htm*.

3. "National Prevalence Study of Methicillin-Resistant Staphylococcus aureus (MRSA) in U.S. Healthcare Facilities," APIC, *www.apic.org* (2006).

4. Ibid.

5. "An APIC Guide to the Elimination of Methicillin-Resistant Staphylococcus Aureus (MRSA) Transmission in Hospital Settings," APIC, *www.apic.org* (2007).

6. Ibid.

7. CDC, *www.cdc.gov*.

8. J.C. Hageman, J.B. Patel, F.C. Tenover, L.C. McDonald, "Investigation And Control Of Vancomycin-Intermediate And -Resistant Staphylococcus Aureus: A Guide For Health Departments And Infection Control Personnel," CDC, *www.cdc.gov/ncidod/dhqp/ar_visavrsa_prevention.html* (2006).

9. Ibid.

10. C. Friedman, S. Callery, A. Jeanes, P. Piaskowski, L. Scott, "International Infection Control Council Best Infection Control Practices for Patients with Extended Spectrum Beta-Lactamase Enterobacteriacae," APIC, *www.apic.org*.

11. "Guidance for Control of Infection with Carbapenem-Resistant or Carbepenemase-Producing Enterobacteriacae in Acute Care Facilities," *Mortality and Morbidity Weekly* 58.10 (2009): 256–260.

12. Ibid.

13. J.D. Siegel, E. Rhinehart, M. Jackson, L. Chiarello, "Management of Multidrug-Resistant Organisms in Healthcare Settings," *American Journal of Infection Control* (2006).

14. G.L. French, "Antimicrobial Resistance in Hospital Flora and Nosocomial Infections," *Hospital Epidemiology and Infection Control,* Third Edition, (Philadelphia: Lippencott Williams & Wilkins, 2004).

15. Ibid.

16. CDC, *www.cdc.gov*.

17. P. Rosenbaum, "Multidrug-Resistant Acinetobacter Baumannii In Long-Term Care Facilities," *APIC Infection Connection* (2008): 1–3.

18. J.P. Flahert, V. Stoser, "Non-Fermentative Gram-Negative Bacilli," *Hospital Epidemiology and Infection Control,* Third Edition, (Philadelphia: Lippencott Williams & Wilkins, 2004).

19. F.W. Vasaly, H.D. Reines, "A Quality Committee's Evaluation of Surgical Intervention for Clostridium Difficile Infection," *AORN Journal* 90 (2009): 192–200.

20. E.R. Dubberke, D.N. Gerding, D. Classes, et al., "Strategies to Prevent Clostridium Difficile Infections in Acute Care Hospitals," *Infection Control and Hospital Epidemiology* 29.1 (2008): S81–S92.

21. *APIC Guide to Elimination of* Clostridium Difficile *in Healthcare Settings,* APIC (2008).

22. Ibid.

23. Ibid.

24. D.N. Gerding, "Pseudomembranous Colitis (Clostridium Difficile)," *APIC Text of Infection Control and Epidemiology,* Second Edition (Washington: Association for Professionals in Infection Control and Epidemiology, Inc., 2005).

25. W.J. Jarvis, J. Schlosser, A.A. Jarvis, R.Y. Chen, "National Point Prevalence of C. Difficile in U.S. Health-care Facility Inpatients," *American Journal of Infection Control* 37 (2009): 263–270.

26. P.D. Levin, M.B. Chir, O. Shatz, et al., "Contamination of Portable X-Ray Equipment with Resistant Bacteria in the ICU," *CHEST* 136 (2009): 426–432.

27. J.D. Siegel, E. Rhinehart, M. Jackson, L. Chiarello, "Management of Multidrug-Resistant Organisms in Healthcare Settings," *American Journal of Infection Control* (2006).

28. Ibid.

CHAPTER 5
Surveillance

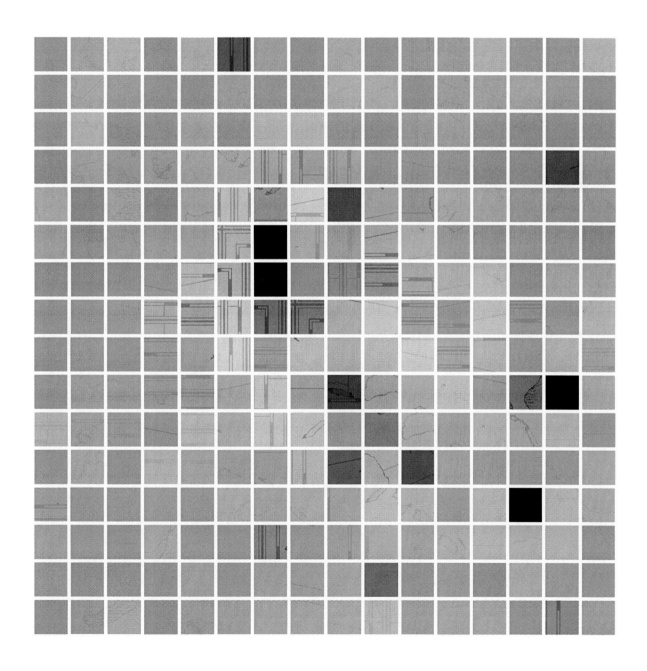

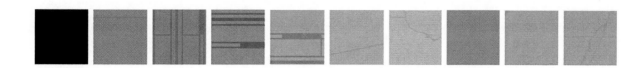

CHAPTER 5

Surveillance

WHAT IS SURVEILLANCE?

Surveillance is an essential part of any infection prevention and control program. The *APIC Text Of Infection Control And Epidemiology* says that "surveillance is a systematic method of collecting, consolidating, and analyzing data concerning the distribution and determinants of a given disease or event, followed by the dissemination of that information to those who can improve the outcomes."[1] With today's goal of zero tolerance for healthcare-associated infections (HAI), surveillance is really the backbone of the program; it serves to identify risk factors for infection, assist in reducing risks, and help monitor the effectiveness of interventions. Surveillance assists the infection preventionist (IP) in identifying clusters or outbreaks of infection, emerging infectious diseases, antimicrobial-resistant organisms, and even bioterrorism events so that infection prevention and control interventions can be put in place. Surveillance is based on sound epidemiological principles and can be used to determine whether our efforts have made a difference in patient outcomes and employee safety.

According to The Joint Commission, surveillance is conducted for multiple purposes, with the ultimate goal of improving the quality of patient safety in healthcare. See Figure 5.1.

FIGURE 5.1 • WHY CONDUCT SURVEILLANCE?

- To determine baseline rates of occurrence of a disease or event

- To detect clusters of infection or outbreaks

- To evaluate prevention and control measures

- To identify potential risk factors for infection

- To observe practice for compliance with recommendations, standards, and facility policies and procedures

- To detect notifiable diseases for reporting to the health department

- To identify organisms of epidemiologic significant such as tuberculosis, hepatitis, and antibiotic-resistant organisms

- To assist risk management in the facility

- To ensure compliance with regulations such as those of the state (e.g., mandatory public reporting), the Occupational Safety and Health Administration, and the Centers for Medicare & Medicaid Services, as well as accrediting agencies such as The Joint Commission

- To assess personnel injuries/illnesses and risk factors

- To detect events such as bioterrorism or emerging infectious diseases

- To provide healthcare workers with real-time data and information on trends in their facility

- To assist with data collection for risk assessments such as those for tuberculosis

ASSESSING RISKS IN YOUR FACILITY

Surveillance is based on your facility's unique risk assessment. Per Joint Commission standards,[2] risks are identified based on the following epidemiological principles:

- Geography, community, and population served

- Care, treatment, and services provided

- Analysis of surveillance data

In the interest of mandatory public reporting of HAIs, many states now have laws that are changing rapidly in terms of what is required for surveillance purposes and reporting to the state. These indicators are of note and must be stated and followed in the written risk assessment. Other critical factors to consider in your risk assessment include the presence of epidemiologically important organisms; high-risk, high-volume, and problem-prone indicators; and assessment of your staff members and patients.

For example, risks will be very different if you work with a population of high-risk women and children versus short-term stay surgical patients or mostly critically ill patients with multiple invasive devices. Enlist the aid of a multidisciplinary group or gather collaborative ideas from the medical staff, hospital leadership, department managers, etc., about who your at-risk populations are in your organization. Don't forget to address staff members as well.

As an example, an ambulatory surgery center may have assessed its risk in the following manner:

- Location in an area prone to hurricanes

- Basically healthy adult population

- High volume of orthopedic procedures, with carpal tunnel repair and endoscopic knee procedures being most frequent

- Past surveillance data show concern for infections after rotator cuff surgery

- Recent increase in procedures in elderly patients with methicillin-resistant *Staphylococcus aureus* infection

- Bloodborne exposures to staff members in the operating room

By noting these risks in a written format, the IP, with assistance from the multidisciplinary group or infection control committee, will be able to prioritize. This will lead to a useful surveillance work plan for the year in which scarce resources and time can be invested in the highest priority items. See Figure 5.2 and 5.3. Through surveillance, the IP is able to demonstrate the quality of care provided by documentation of the outcomes. After a comprehensive infection control risk assessment, the IP will be able to lay out a written plan to serve as the foundation for the surveillance program. Each organization's surveillance program will be unique for that organization and should be evaluated at least annually. At that time, any surveillance outcome indicators as well as process indicators (see Figure 5.4) that have remained stable and unchanged over time may be considered for discontinuation in favor of addressing those with higher priority or newer challenges.

FIGURE 5.2 •SAMPLE RISK ASSESSMENT FOR AMBULATORY SURGERY CENTERS

Patient/Employee Population	Service Provided	Identified Risk	Level of Risk	Strategies for Prevention
1. Healthy adults	Rotator cuff surgery	Surgical site infections	Problem prone	Surveillance, reporting, observing technique in the operating room, traffic control
2. Healthy adults	Knee scopes	Mandatory reporting required by the state	Low risk	Surveillance of procedure post discharge by letters to surgeons, analyze and feed back the data to individual surgeons and surgical staff members
3. Healthy adults	Carpal tunnel repairs	Potential for surgical site infection	High volume	Surveillance of procedure post discharge by letters to surgeons, analyze and feed back the data to individual surgeons and surgical staff members
4. Bloodborne exposures among the operating room staff	Mainly due to passing instruments in the operating room	Risk to employees of blood-borne diseases	High risk	Compliance with the bloodborne pathogens standard and sharps safety, compliance with hepatitis B vaccine, trial use of neutral zone in the operating room, staff education on the above and reporting of exposures as soon as possible
5. Elderly patients from community and nursing homes	Orthopedic surgery	MRSA infection (upon admission)	High risk, problem prone; epidemiologically important organism	Consider potential preoperative screening for MRSA on all nursing home patients, use pop-up screens, monitor compliance with hand hygiene and standard precautions
6. Mainly healthy adults	Ambulatory surgery	Hurricane-prone area	High risk	Include hurricane planning in disaster management, ensure provision of the alcohol hand gels and scrubs and alternative sources for water and sterile water, consider a staffing plan

FIGURE 5.3 • RISK ASSESSMENT*

Patient/Employee Population	Service Provided	Identified Risk	Level of Risk**	Strategies for Prevention
1.				
2.				
3.				
4.				
5.				
6.				

* Risks based on order of priority
** Level of risk: Examples include high volume, high risk, problem prone, mandatory reporting required by state, epidemiological-important organisms, etc.

FIGURE 5.4 • SURVEILLANCE INDICATORS

Indicator	Definition	Example
Outcome	Result of healthcare or performance	Infection, injury, patient satisfaction (e.g., ventilator-associated pneumonia rate)
Process	Series of steps to achieve an outcome	Immunization, compliance with a specific bundle of care, etc.

STEPS OF SURVEILLANCE

A wonderful resource for new and seasoned IPs to refer to periodically is the "2007 Recommended Practices For Surveillance: Association For Professionals In Infection Control And Epidemiology (APIC), Inc."[3] According to this article, the seven recommended steps of surveillance are:

1. Assess the population

2. Select the outcomes or processes for surveillance

3. Use written surveillance definitions

4. Collect surveillance data

5. Calculate and analyze rates of infection

6. Apply risk stratification

7. Report and use surveillance information

Let's discuss each one and how they apply to *your* program.

Step 1: Assess the population

This is what we have mentioned in the risk assessment. Who is your population? What types of patients do you see? What services do you provide? Who are your high-volume patients? What are your high-volume procedures? What are your high-risk or problem-prone areas? What community concerns are there? How about your organization's strategic plan? Have you addressed those issues (e.g., if your facility wants to become a center of cardiac surgery excellence, what should you survey?). You can use many in-house resources to assist you in this area, such as medical records, financial reports, risk management reports, operating room logs, employee health reports, etc. Don't forget to use the expertise of your team members as well.

Step 2: Select the outcomes or processes for surveillance

Along with assessing the population, the IP needs to simultaneously select what to survey. (See Figure 5.4 for guidance). Which indicators are most relevant to your organization? What are your most frequent concerns? Which areas give you the most problems or offer the most chance for prevention? Which meet your customers' needs, including those of leadership? Perhaps you will follow all coronary artery bypass procedures since leadership wants this to be a center of excellence for your organization. Also, because you have read recent literature and find that there is much lacking in your ventilator-associated pneumonia (VAP) prevention program, you could elect

THE INFECTION PREVENTION HANDBOOK |

to follow VAPs (high risk and opportunity for prevention) in these same patients simultaneously or in all ICUs. Don't forget to also select those areas that are required for mandatory reporting by your state, if applicable. You must follow those indicators. Choose several indicators to follow, but don't go overboard. None of us have unlimited resources. You don't want to spend all your time performing surveillance and collecting data. You will need to address the issues you find from the surveillance data, such as through education, creation of new policies and procedure, and formation of teams. Direct you resources toward your highest-ranked priorities, but don't forget to reassess your priorities at least annually. Priorities change, other issues arise, and some indicators may be resolved and no longer need to be surveyed. You will find that having a prioritized plan to follow will help keep you on track with your concerns and won't allow you to become sidetracked.

Step 3: Use written surveillance definitions

Definitions will help you ensure more precise surveillance data. The definitions should be standardized so that infection is interpreted consistently at all times. Let's take the example of the McGeer Long-Term Care Definitions,[4] which have been in use for years.

McGeer Long-Term Care Definitions

The definition of a urinary infection from these written definitions is as follows:

One of the following criteria must be met:

1. *The resident does not have an indwelling urinary catheter and has at least three of the following signs and symptoms: (a) fever (greater than or equal to 38°C) or chills, (b) new or increased burning pain on urination or frequency or urgency, (c) new flank or suprapubic pain or tenderness, (d) change in character of urine,* (e) worsening of mental or functional status (may be new or increased incontinence)*

2. *The resident has an indwelling catheter and has at least two of the following signs or symptoms: (a) fever (great than or equal to 38°C) or chills, (b) new flank or suprapubic pain or tenderness, (c) change in character of urine,* and/or (d) worsening of mental or functional status*

It should be noted that urine culture results are not included in the criteria. However, if an appropriately collected and processed urine specimen was sent and if the resident was not taking antibiotics at the time, then the culture must be reported as either positive or contaminated. Because the most common occult infectious source of fever in catheterized residents is the urinary tract, the combination of fever and worsening mental or functional status in such residents meets the criteria for a urinary tract infection. However, particular care should be taken to rule out other causes of these symptoms. If a catheterized resident with only fever and worsening mental or functional status meets the criteria for infection at a site other than the urinary tract, only the diagnosis of infection at this other site should be made.

*Change in character may be clinical (e.g., new bloody urine, foul smell, or amount of sediment) or as reported by the laboratory (new pyuria or microscopic hematuria). For laboratory changes, this means that a previous urinalysis must have been negative.[5]

Compare this to APIC's Home Care Definitions for urinary tract infection.[6]

APIC's Home Care Definitions

The definition of a urinary infection from these written definitions is as follows:

Symptomatic UTIs can occur without prior instrumentation (e.g., intermittent catheterization), but this is rare.

Catheter-associated UTIs are associated with instrumentation of the patient's urinary tract prior to onset. To associate these infections with an indwelling urinary catheter requires presence of an indwelling urinary catheter at the time of or within seven days before the onset of the symptomatic UTI.

Symptomatic and catheter-associated UTIs must meet one of the following criteria:

> 1. *Two of the following four signs or symptoms:*
>   a. *Fever **OR** chills with no other external urinary source noted*
>   b. *Flank pain, **OR** suprapubic pain, **OR** tenderness, **OR** frequency, **OR** urgency*

   c. Worsening of mental **OR** functional status

   d. Changes in urine character (e.g., new bloody urine, foul odor, increased sediment) **AND** urinalysis or culture is not done

2. One of the following two signs or symptoms:

   a. Fever **OR** chills

   b. Flank pain, **OR** suprapubic pain, **OR** tenderness, **AND** both bacteriuria (determined by a positive urine culture for a potential pathogen or a positive nitrite assay by dipstick) and pyuria (determined by 10 or more wbc/hpf on urinalysis or positive leukocyte esterase assay by dipstick)

Note: Asymptomatic UTIs are not included in these definitions.

If we use the example of an 80-year-old female with a Foley catheter who is bedridden in her home and develops chills and bacteriuria and pyuria on urinalysis, home care definitions would qualify this patient as having an HAI. However, if the long-term definitions were used for surveillance purposes, the patient would not qualify as having a healthcare-associated UTI. It is easy to understand from the two sets of different definitions used above how critical it is to have written definitions approved by the Infection Prevention and Control Committee (or like committee) to ensure consistency in surveillance data over time.[7]

Also note that if the definitions change (e.g., the home care agency has been using the long-term care definitions but now has agreed to switch to the newer home care definitions), then the data after the use of the new definitions is incomparable to the previous data.

Step 4: Collect surveillance data

Trained personnel should collect and manage the data collected. Many facilities are still collecting data manually, but the IP should collaborate with the information technology department to determine what's available in terms of resources to support surveillance. There is also commercially available software to scan through large amounts of data and increase the efficiency of surveillance.[8] Using only passively obtained data, such as having the unit nurses call the IP when a patient has an infection, will usually result in underreporting of infections. Administrative data, such as that used by hospital coders,[9] are not valid or reliable for epidemiological purposes. The

IP should collect data from many sources, such as from inpatient and outpatients charts, operating room logs and databases, and caregivers, as well as from laboratory, radiology, and pharmacy. However, only collect data that will be used. A surveillance worksheet for each initiative (e.g., urinary tract infection) and each patient is very useful and can be developed simply by listing the patient demographics and date of admission along with specific surveillance definitions of infections (check which ones apply), and date of occurrence. These worksheets can then be compiled into line lists (see Figure 5.5 as an example).

FIGURE 5.5 • LINE LISTING EXAMPLE

Methicillin-resistant *Staphylococcus aureus* (MRSA): YEAR

Doctor	Patient	Medical Record #	Admission Date	Room	Diagnosis	Culture Site/Date	Medicine	Present on Admission/ Hospital-Acquired Infection	Comments

Step 5: Calculate and analyze rates of infection

Presenting raw data on infections and numbers of infections may be misleading. The data should be studied, analyzed, and presented in numerical terms such as rates, ratios, and proportions. Prior to collection of data, determine what you wish to measure. Rates (ratios and proportions) are fractions. The numerator (top number) is the number of events (such as infections) detected during the time period studied and the denominator (bottom number) is the population at risk. For example, if you are following coronary artery bypass grafts (CABG), the numerator would be the number of CABGs infected divided by the total number of CABGs performed for the month or quarter (denominator). If the denominator is too small, rates may appear unusually high; therefore, calculations should possibly be performed less frequently (e.g., every six months or annually). This is an example of an outcome.

Processes are also measured at times. For example, instead of measuring VAP rates, you could choose to measure compliance with the VAP bundle of interventions per the Institute for Healthcare Improvement. Since the bundle is meant to be implemented as a whole and not in a piecemeal fashion, any noncompliance in the checklist (Table 5.2) for one patient would mean that care is noncompliant (all or none). However, by looking at individual criteria, such as hand hygiene or use of maximal sterile barriers for insertion, you can determine where specific problems lie in performing the interventions required to prevent central line–associated bloodstream infections. In this case, the numerator would be the number of patients observed with ALL five elements of the central line bundle compliant divided by the number with central lines on the day of the observations (denominator).

Step 6: Apply risk stratification

Every individual in a group or population is not at the same level of risk for infection. For example, newborns in a normal weight range are less at risk than those who are extremely underweight. Therefore, if we can stratify (or group) them by weight classifications, such as > 2500 g, 1501–2500 g, 1110–1500 g, 751–1000 g, < 750 g, we would expect the tiniest of infants to have the highest risk of infection. Following the same logic, "clean" surgeries (an uninfected operative wound in which no inflammation is encountered and the respiratory, alimentary, genital, or uninfected urinary tract is not entered) should have a lower risk of infection than "dirty" surgeries (old traumatic wounds with retained devitalized tissue and those that involve existing clinical infection or perforated viscera).[10]

By grouping or risk-stratifying patients in this manner, more meaningful and accurate comparisons of the data can be made over time. For some populations, risk stratification may be impossible; however, one caveat holds true: The subpopulation data must be large enough to be statistically meaningful.

Step 7: Report and use surveillance information

Sharing the analyzed data with those in leadership and those who can affect change is a powerful force. Doing so has proven time and again to improve performance. With whom and how frequently the data should be shared should be noted in your infection prevention and control plan. The data should be presented on an ongoing basis in user-friendly formats such as tables, pie chart, graphs, along with written analysis.

Note: For surveillance data to be compared internally in the facility or externally, comparisons are valid ONLY if:

- Surveillance intensity is consistent (e.g., twice per week)

- Similar data collection methods are used

- The same written surveillance definitions are used

- Differences in population are addressed

- Data are stratified, as appropriate

Automated surveillance through data mining (discovering trends and relationships for predictions among large amounts of data and query-based data management (i.e., a process that does not seek patterns independently but does require user input) can free the IP to spend time on prevention instead of realms of paperwork with manual surveillance. The Association for Professionals in Prevention Control and Epidemiology has created a position paper on surveillance technologies and also has an assessment tool to help facilities select an appropriate system.[11]

CONCLUSION

Surveillance is the cornerstone of a program that is effective in infection prevention and control. Surveillance allows us to determine whether we are reaching excellence in infection prevention as we strive for zero tolerance, or whether our efforts need to be rerouted or increased. Infection prevention and control programs would do well to incorporate automated surveillance whenever possible in their programs to streamline the process and use fewer manpower hours on this activity in order to spend time where our efforts can truly make a difference: education, performance improvement, and prevention.

REFERENCES

1. R. Carrico, *APIC Text Of Infection Control And Epidemiology,* Second Edition, (Washington, DC: Association for Professionals in Infection Control and Epidemiology, 2005), 3–18, *www.apic.org.*

2. The Joint Commission, *2009 Comprehensive Accreditation Manual for Hospital Accreditation, www. jointcommission.org.*

3. T.B. Lee, O.G. Montgomery, J. Marx, R.N. Olmsted, W.E. Scheckler, "Recommended Practices For Surveillance: Association For Professionals In Infection Control And Epidemiology, (APIC), Inc.," *American Journal Infection Control* 35 (2007): 427–440.

4. A. McGeer, B. Campbell, T.G. Emori, et al., "Definitions Of Infections For Surveillance In Long-Term Care Facilities," *American Journal of Infection Control,* 19 (1991): 1–7.

5. Ibid

6. APIC, *HICPAC Surveillance Definitions for Home Health Care and Home Hospice Infections*, February, 2008, *www.apic.org.*

7. Ibid.

8. APIC, *Surveillance Technology Resources, www.apic.org.*

9. E.R. Sherman, K.H. Heydon, K.H. St. John, E. Tezner, S.L. Rettig, S.K. Alexander, et al., "Administrative Data Fail to Accurately Identify Cases of Healthcare-Associated Infection," *Infection Control Hospital Epidemiology* 27 (2006): 332–337.

10. A.J. Mangram, T.C. Horan, M.L. Pearson, L.C. Silver, W.R. Jarvis, CDC Guideline for Prevention of Surgical Site Infection," *Infection Control Hospital Epidemiology* 20 (1999): 247–278.

11. "Position Paper: The Importance of Surveillance Technologies in the Prevention of Healthcare-Associated Infections HAIS)," APIC, *www.apic.org.*

The Infection Prevention and Control Plan

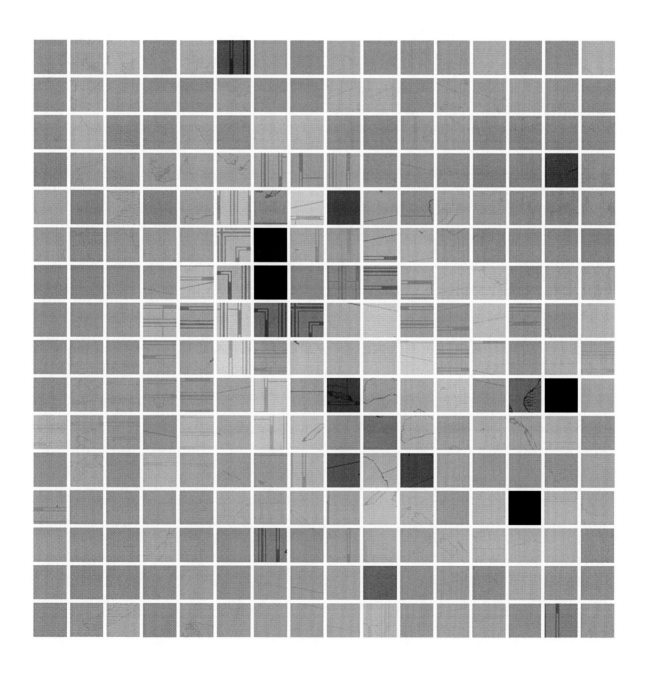

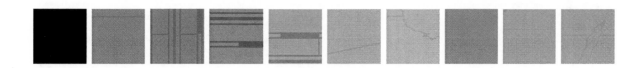

The Infection Prevention and Control Plan

WHY IS A PLAN NECESSARY?

Every business needs a plan. The same holds true for the business of infection prevention and control. In its standards, The Joint Commission states that an organization must have an infection prevention and control plan. Without a plan, we don't know in which direction to go. A plan paints a picture in broad strokes of our facility and what we hope to accomplish for the year. Before our plan is complete, our risk assessment should already be completed, and the plan should take into account the geography, community, and population served; care, treatment, and services provided at our organization; and analysis of surveillance data in addition to any mandatory reporting requirements of our state. Specifically, it includes a written description of the planned activities, including surveillance, used to reduce or eliminate the risk of infection. A written plan will guide our work as we move forward in our program each year. The plan is always dynamic and should never remain exactly the same from year to year. New issues arise, new infectious disease threats must be handled, and facilities expand and grow into alternative care sites in the community. The challenges are many. Our plan will help us stay on track and focused on what we must accomplish to reduce infections in our patients and staff members.

WHAT'S INCLUDED IN THE PLAN?

Infection control plans will vary based on the organization and its needs, as well as regulatory and accreditation requirements. It may be helpful to write your plan in an outline and fill in the blanks afterward. (See Figure 6.1 as a reference.) Your bloodborne plan and tuberculosis plan may be included here or as separate documents.

DOES IT WORK?

Our most important task is evaluating the plan at least annually or more often if risks change significantly (such as adding a new service like bronchoscopy). Have you made an impact in the care of patients and health of employees? Are there other strategies you can employ and evaluate? Be sure to continue surveillance so you can determine whether you indeed made a difference in lowering infection rates or bettering practices of care. The Joint Commission requires that the infection preventionist (IP) evaluate the effectiveness of the infection control and prevention plan and use this information to revise the plan as needed. To view another IP's plan, risk assessment, evaluation of the plan, and revision of the plan, see Figure 6.2.

FIGURE 6.1 • OUTLINE OF AN INFECTION PREVENTION AND CONTROL PLAN

A. Infection prevention and control department:
1. Organizationwide
2. Personnel and qualifications including support staff members
3. Resources (e.g., equipment, computers, references, training opportunities)
4. Authority
5. IP professional activities

B. Risk assessment:
1. Facility size and type; scope of care, service, procedures, and treatment provided; issues from surveillance data; and geography and community
2. Patient population
3. Types of personnel
4. Description of prioritized risks to target at this facility this year:
   a. First priority _____
   b. _____
   c. _____
   d. _____
   e. _____
   f. _____
   g. _____
   h. _____

C. Goals and objectives (describe broad goals and list a measurable objective for each goal):
   a. Goal: _____
      Objective: _____
   b. Goal: _____
      Objective: _____
   c. Goal: _____
      Objective: _____
   d. Goal: _____
      Objective: _____
   e. Goal: _____
      Objective: _____
   f. Goal: _____
      Objective: _____
   g. Goal: _____
      Objective: _____
   h. Goal: _____
      Objective: _____

FIGURE 6.1 • OUTLINE OF AN INFECTION PREVENTION AND CONTROL PLAN (CONT.)

D. Strategies to reduce the risk for each objective (include actions associated with procedures, equipment, and devices; policies and procedures based on current guidelines and regulations; isolation; investigation of outbreaks; employee health screening; work restriction; employee education; environmental issues, such as routine rounds and handling of infectious wastes; special issues, such as renovation and construction; and education and training offered, etc.)

Objective a: _____

Objective b: _____

Objective c: _____

Objective d: _____

Objective e: _____

Objective f: _____

Objective g: _____

Objective h: _____

E. Surveillance plan:

    a. Assessment of risks for your specific patients and staff members:

_____

_____

_____

    b. Description of indicators to monitor (include outcomes and processes):

_____

_____

_____

    c. Antibiogram:

_____

_____

_____

    d. Reporting of surveillance data (include to whom, how often, and required reports of infectious diseases to public health department):

_____

_____

_____

    e. Outbreaks:

_____

_____

_____

FIGURE 6.1 • OUTLINE OF AN INFECTION PREVENTION AND CONTROL PLAN (CONT.)

F. **Performance improvement projects** (planned or ongoing):

_____

_____

_____

_____

_____

_____

G. **Emergency management planning:**

_____

_____

_____

_____

_____

_____

H. **Evaluation process** (evaluate each goal and objective as well as staffing and support for your department, such as nonpersonnel resources):

a. _____

_____

_____

b. _____

_____

_____

c. _____

_____

_____

d. _____

_____

_____

e. _____

_____

_____

f. _____

_____

_____

g. _____

_____

_____

Reprinted with permission from Libby Chinnes, RN, BSN, CIC; IC Solutions, LLC.

FIGURE 6.2 • SAMPLE CORE PROGRAM EVALUATION FOR 2006			
2005 Plan	**Do**	**Check**	**Act/Plan for 2006**
Hand hygiene			
Complete conversion and evaluate function-ality of new dispenser	Replaced alcohol hand wash dispenser with an improved design	Improved function with new dispensers	Quarterly hand hygiene to be monitored in select areas with ongoing education
When the Centers for Medicare & Medic-aid Services gives approval, install dispensers in hallways as appropriate	General orientation focused on hand hygiene, including giving out letter opener with hand hygiene logo		General orientation to continue focus on hand hygiene
Continue education initiative to promote proper hand hygiene	Ongoing education of staff members about the use of alcohol products		
Safety devices			
Continue to evaluate exposure data	Regional and local historical data reviewed	Recommendation made to products committee to trial different protected IV catheter/butterflies	• Change safety IV products if staff members evalua-tion indicates • Continue to evaluate safety data
		Exposure occurrences have doubled at hospital	Explore the market for safety syringes and suture needles
		Lab trialing two different safety butter-fly devices in the fourth quarter of 2005	
		Trial of passive IV catheter device in December 2005	

FIGURE 6.2 • SAMPLE CORE PROGRAM EVALUATION FOR 2006 (CONT.)			
2005 Plan	**Do**	**Check**	**Act/Plan for 2006**
Policy review			
Update policies appropriately as guidelines are published	Reviewed and placed in an online format	Creutzfeldt-Jakob Disease (CJD) policy completed collaboratively with surgery and infection control	Meet guidelines for timely policy review Continue education regarding CJD policy
Policies are online in 2005		Education in process in the fourth quarter of 2005	Assess for best practice
		Annual review of the exposure control plan and tuberculosis control (required by the Occupational Safety and Health Administration)	
		Process complete	
Purified protein derivative (PPD) testing			
Continue annual PPD testing program	Screening performed with 100% compliance	No conversions	Continue in 2006
Tuberculosis cases			
	One case identified	Follow-up to exposure performed—no conversions	Continue to monitor in 2006
Influenza			
Continue the vaccine program for employees and volunteers	Vaccine offered free	43% of staff members received influenza vaccine. National average is 36%.	Continue in 2006
			Educate to promote vaccination for the 2005–2006 season

FIGURE 6.2 • SAMPLE CORE PROGRAM EVALUATION FOR 2006 (CONT.)			
2005 Plan	**Do**	**Check**	**Act/Plan for 2006**
Education			
Participate in mandatory/competency education for various departments in 2005	Revised mandatory computer-based infection control education modules	Complete	Participate in education for various departments in 2006
Use general orientation to educate 100% of employees about hand hygiene	Presented content at mandatory nursing sessions regarding identified issues with isolation procedures and communication issues		Continue assessment of isolation practice and communication
Antibiograms			
Review 2004 and previous years' antibiogram		Antibiograms placed	Review 2005 antibiogram and distribute for medical staff members
Copies placed in dictation areas			
Surgical site infection (SSI)			
Targeted surveillance		Hospital rates within National Nosocomial Infection Surveillance System/National Healthcare Safety Network rates	Continue monitoring procedures approved for the 2006 surveillance plan
Perform surveillance on targeted procedures approved by the physical therapy/infection control committee		Standing orders implemented and improved consistency	Continue monitoring surgical infection prevention project procedures approved for 2006: • Hip arthroplasty • Knee arthroplasty • Vascular surgery • Hysterectomy • Colon procedures
Prophylaxis and SSI prevention		Decreased postoperative doses in total hip/knee to ensure 24-hour discontinuation	Await publication of the revised medical letter with recommendations for colon surgery prophylaxis and focus on implementation

FIGURE 6.2 • SAMPLE CORE PROGRAM EVALUATION FOR 2006 (CONT.)			
2005 Plan	**Do**	**Check**	**Act/Plan for 2006**
Surgical site infection (SSI) (cont.)			
Monitor timing in cases selected in the 2004 surveillance plan		Increased ancef antibiotic dosing in total knee population Implemented weight-based ancef dosing in total hip population and vancomycin dosing for total knee replacement and total hip replacement Worked toward no-razor preps Implemented educa-tion program with patients about no-razor shaving of operative area 72 hours prior to surgery	Continue working on antibiotic selection, timing, and discontinuation
		Formulated a task force to look at status of deep venous thrombosis (DVT) prophylaxis, hypother-mia, vent bundling, beta-blocker, and surgical population	Continue task force efforts
ICU			
Monitor ventilator-associated pneumonia	Surveillance performed	2005: 0 per 1,000 vent days 2004: 289 per 1,000 vent days 2003: 446 per 1,000 vent days 2002: 512 per 1,000 vent days Implemented in ICU	Continue to monitor

FIGURE 6.2 • SAMPLE CORE PROGRAM EVALUATION FOR 2006 (CONT.)			
2005 Plan	**Do**	**Check**	**Act/Plan for 2006**
ICU (Cont.)			
Meet with the ICU to discuss ventilator bundles (head of bed elevated 30°, DVT prophylaxis, sedation vacation, assessment for extubation readiness, glucose monitoring)	Bundling orders completed and implemented	Inconsistent use of bundling; vent bundling orders included into ICU order set to promote use	Continue to monitor
Monitor bacteremias associated with central lines (ICU and housewide)	Surveillance performed	ICU 2005: 50 per 1,000 line days (line day data compromised) 2004: 0 per 1,000 days 2003: 37 per 1,000 line days 2002: 54 per 1,000 line days	Monitor specific lines per the 2005 surveillance plan
Work with the ICU to review central line bundles	Policies revised Ongoing education Central line cart stocked with all supplies Kits stocked with chloraprep	Product issues still identified	Infection control to make recommendation to regional products regarding product issues
Develop housewide monitoring of central line insertion	Central line monitor implemented	Monitor reflects 100% compliance in radiology improvement noted housewide	Continue to work with vendors to receive products with appropriate components Continue monitoring and education efforts with physicians and staff members
Multidrug-resistant organisms/outbreaks and significant infections			
VRE	Monitor the number of cases	2001: 2 2002: 3 2003: 6 2004: 3 2005: 6	Continue to monitor
MRSA		Rate of community-acquired MRSA found to be significantly higher than nosocomial (86% vs. 14% of all MRSA cultures)	Continue to monitor Share data and educational information with the ED

FIGURE 6.2 • SAMPLE CORE PROGRAM EVALUATION FOR 2006 (CONT.)			
2005 Plan	**Do**	**Check**	**Act/Plan for 2006**
Best practice/policy development			
	Specialists from all acute care sites meet monthly to review policy and to practice and respond to current healthcare concerns/ issues/guidelines		Continue IC meetings
	Participated in Greater Cincinnati Health Council Infection Control Group to discuss issues relative to community: MRSA, isolation, bioterrorism, influenza	Visitor restrictions during influenza season implemented in cooperation with all area hospitals	Continue to participate in Greater Cincinnati Health Council Infec- tion Control Group
	Implemented chlora- prep for peripheral IV therapy	Done	Continue to meet quarterly
Pneumococcal vaccine			
Continue pneumococcal screening criteria in admission process	Pneumococcal screen- ing criteria incorpo- rated into admission process Charts of eligible patients stickered for physician management	Increase from 48% in 2003 to 72% in 2004	Continue
Work with the disaster committee to develop an effective plan to manage an influx of infectious patients	Policy generated and approved by the safety committee Format fits into the disaster plan		Evaluate plan and revise detail
Identified concerns: Monitor compliance with transmission- based precautions and communication of precautions	Monitoring performed Deficiencies addressed as found Major education focus in mandatory nursing education days		Continue to monitor
Reporting: Ensure compliance with reporting regula- tions of communicable diseases in Ohio		Reports made in compliance with regulations	Continue
Construction: Complete construction risk assessments as projects are planned		Assessments complet- ed with the safety director	Continue

FIGURE 6.2 • SAMPLE CORE PROGRAM EVALUATION FOR 2006 (CONT.)

Assessment of services and risk

Hospital X is a suburban hospital serving both suburban and rural areas. Services provided include:

- Sixty med-surg beds

- A 12-bed medical-surgical ICU

- Thirty adult behavioral medicine beds

- Thirty-six thousand emergency visits per year

- Wound care center

- Outpatient chemo/endo/bronch

Populations served are:

- Forty percent Medicare

- Twenty-eight percent Medicaid/self-pay

- Adult inpatient population

- Emergency department: 20% pediatric

High risk

- Bacteremia associated with central lines

- Ventilator-associated pneumonia

- Surgical site infection

High volume

- Surgical population

- Emergency department visits

Problem prone

- Total knee replacements

Improvement needed

- Antibiotic prophylaxis administration

- Appropriate insertion/care of central lines

FIGURE 6.2 • SAMPLE CORE PROGRAM EVALUATION FOR 2006 (CONT.)

Assessment of services and risk (Cont.)

For each prioritized risk, identify goals, strategies, responsible person, time frame, and evaluation of effectiveness.

Priority risk	Goals	Strategies	Implementation		
			Responsible person	*Time frame*	*Method and evaluation of effectiveness*
Bacteremia associated with central lines	Accomplish 95% compliance (outside radiology) with best practice guidelines for central lines	Monitor insertion of central lines Physician education Staff member education Physician-to-physician discussion	Infection control specialists Physicians Nursing staff members	Ongoing from 2005 Calculate monthly	Central line insertion monitor Bacteremia surveillance
Surgical site infection	Maintain current rates or decrease	Weekly assessment of prophylaxis data Monthly surgical site infection surveillance mailer Temperature monitoring of surgical patients	IC specialists Surgeons Department of surgery	Ongoing from 2005 Calculate monthly	SSI surveillance Prophylaxis surveillance
Maintain core key aspects of an effective, fluid infection control program	Maintain core program elements	See the act/plan column in annual evaluation above	Infection control specialists All staff members Employee health	Ongoing from 2005	Ongoing assessment of act/plan above Assessment of surveillance data Assessment of exposure data

Signature	Date	
		Infection control chair
		Infection control specialist
		Quality director
		Safety officer
		Vice president of patient care services

Reprinted with permission from Rosie Fardo.

Monitoring, Reporting, and Performance Improvement

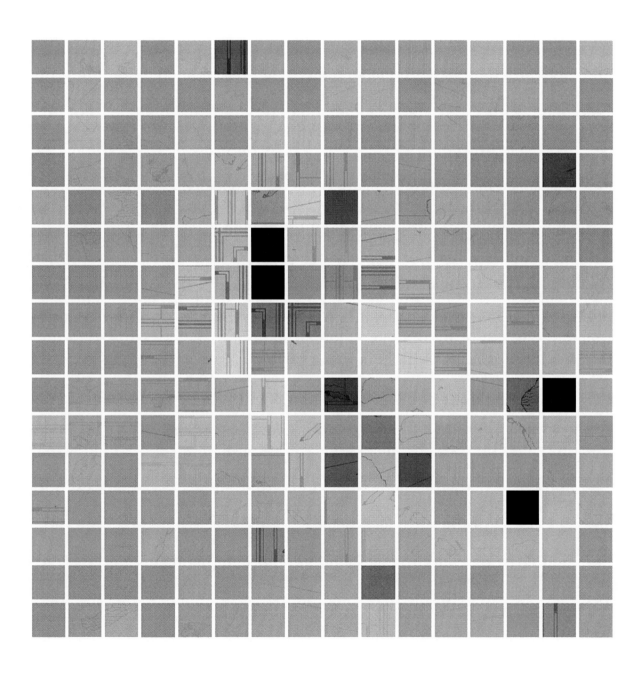

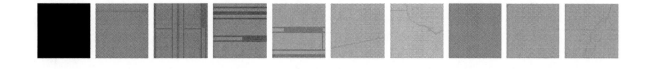

Monitoring, Reporting, and Performance Improvement

MONITORING AND MEASURING

The goal of an infection prevention and control program is to reduce the risk of acquisition and transmission of healthcare-associated infections (HAI). Without monitoring and measuring trends, neither the IP nor the facility will truly know whether success has been reached. It is important to remember to monitor outcomes *and* processes relating to patients *and* staff members. Analyze the information, compare it to previous periods, look for clusters or outbreaks, and put it in a meaningful format for those who can effect change, such as clinicians and providers at the bedside. A sample of processes and outcomes connected with central line–associated bacteremias and ventilator-associated pneumonias is shown in Figure 7.1.

For example, if you demonstrate that your central line–associated infection rate is rising, you can begin to look at bedside practice with central lines or use the bundle measures you are monitoring on an ongoing basis. Showing the staff members a percentage of the total bundle compliance as well as each item of the bundle is an excellent way to tease out deficiencies in practice. You can add this to the outcome data you have (central line–associated bacteremia infection rate) and present this to the staff members regularly and in real time as much as possible. See Figures 7.1 and 7.2 for bundling tools and Figure 7.3 for a tool on hand hygiene monitoring.

FIGURE 7.1 • MONITORING OUTCOMES AND PROCESSES

How to monitor outcomes	How to monitor processes
Central line–associated bloodstream infection (CLABSI) rate per 1,000 line days: Total number of CLABSI cases x 1,000 Number of catheter days	Central line bundle compliance: Number of patients with all five elements of the central line bundle x 100 Number of patients with central lines on the day of the sample
Ventilator-associated pneumonia (VAP) rate per 1,000 line days: Total number of VAP cases x 1,000 Number of ventilator days	VAP bundle compliance: Number of patients with all five elements of VAP bundle x 100 Number of patients with ventilators on the day of the sample

Source: Reprinted with permission from the *5 Million Lives Campaign. Getting Started Kit: Prevent Ventilator-Associated Pneumonia How-to Guide* and the *Prevent Central Line Infections How-to Guide* Cambridge, MA: Institute for Healthcare Improvement; 2008. (Available at *www.ihi.org.*)

FIGURE 7.2 • CENTRAL LINE BUNDLE MONITORING TOOL

Date: _____

Initials: _____

Bundle measure	Pt 1		Pt 2		Pt 3		Pt 4		Pt 5		Comments
Check (√)	Y	N	Y	N	Y	N	Y	N	Y	N	
Hand hygiene											
Maximal barrier precautions upon insertion											
Chlorhexidine skin antisepsis											
Optimal catheter site selection, with avoidance of the femoral vein for central venous access in adult patients											
Daily review of line necessity, with prompt removal of unnecessary lines											

Source: Reprinted with permission from the *5 Million Lives Campaign. Getting Started Kit: Prevent Ventilator-Associated Pneumonia How-to Guide* and the *Prevent Central Line Infections How-to Guide* Cambridge, MA: Institute for Healthcare Improvement; 2008. (Available at *www.ihi.org.*)

FIGURE 7.3 • VAP BUNDLE MONITORING TOOL

Date: _____

Initials: _____

VAP bundle measure	Pt 1		Pt 2		Pt 3		Pt 4		Pt 5		Comments
Check (√)	Y	N	Y	N	Y	N	Y	N	Y	N	
Elevate HOB 30°–45°											
Daily sedation vacation											
Daily assessment of readiness to extubate											
Peptic ulcer disease prophylaxis											
Deep vein thrombosis prophylaxis, unless contraindicated											

Source: Reprinted with permission from the *5 Million Lives Campaign. Getting Started Kit: Prevent Ventilator-Associated Pneumonia How-to Guide* and the *Prevent Central Line Infections How-to Guide* Cambridge, MA: Institute for Healthcare Improvement; 2008. (Available at *www.ihi.org*.)

Remember compliance can be measured in many ways. For example, consider compliance with hand hygiene, which may be measured through observations, volume of product used, or patient satisfaction surveys (or several of these methods). To compare your findings with those of others, you must use the same definitions of terms, same calculation, same frequency, etc. A wonderful reference for in-depth monitoring of hand hygiene compliance and resource tools is *Measuring Hand Hygiene Adherence: Overcoming the Challenges* (2009) by The Joint Commission *(www. jointcommission.org)*. For an example of a hand hygiene tool, see Figure 7.4.

FIGURE 7.4 • INFECTION CONTROL HAND HYGIENE MONITOR

Instructions:

Each observer should collect data on 20 hand washing observations per month.

Observations are to be made on any healthcare workers either before or after patient care.

Observations may be performed on the same day or on different days and/or different shifts. Observations may be made on the same patient receiving care from multiple care workers.

Discipline:

Respiratory=RT, Unit Tech=UT, Physical Therapy=PT, Radiology=XR, Transport=T, Environmental=E, Physician=MD, RN/LPN=N

Unit: _____

Month/Year (mm/yy) ____ / ____	1	2	3	4	5	6	7	8	9	10	11	12	13	14	15	16	17	18	19	20
Discipline—see above																				
Before Care Hand washing (Y,N)																				
Before Care Alcohol Gel (Y,N)																				
After Care Hand washing (Y,N)																				
After Care Alcohol Gel (Y,N)																				

Process:

Alcohol Base Rub

1. Product applied to palm of one hand and hands rubbed together
2. All surfaces of hand and fingers are covered
3. Hands and fingers rubbed until dry

Soap and Water

1. Wet hands with water first
2. Product applied to hands and hands rubbed together for >=15 seconds
3. All surfaces of hand and fingers covered
4. Rinse hands with water and dry thoroughly with a paper towel
5. Use paper towel to turn of water faucet (if hand operated)

Source: Reprinted with permission from Linda Greene.

Examples of other measures that can be monitored for performance improvement include, but are not limited to:

- Percentage of staff members compliant with influenza vaccine = number of staff members who received vaccine ÷ number of eligible staff members x 100

- Percentage of staff members compliant with hand hygiene = number of hand hygiene compliance acts when the opportunity existed ÷ total number of hand hygiene opportunities x 100

- *Clostridium difficile* rate per 1,000 patient days = number of healthcare-associated *Clostridium difficile* cases for a given time period ÷ total number of patient days for same time period x 1,000

- HAI/colonization rate for methicillin-resistant *Staphylococcus aureus* (MRSA) per 1,000 patient days = number cases of HAI /colonization with MRSA for given time period ÷ number of patient days for same time period x 1,000

The Centers for Disease Control and Prevention's National Healthcare Safety Network (*www.cdc.gov/nhsn/psc.html*) compiles data from many facilities, including outpatient centers. Although our goal is always zero tolerance for any HAI, we can benchmark against the National Healthcare Safety Network data if we use the same protocols to strive for lower infection rates in our facilities.

PERFORMANCE IMPROVEMENT

Now that you have measured some aspects of the quality of care in your facility, how do you go about improving them? First of all, don't let your surveillance and reports merely go to committees or sit on your desk to be filed away. Share the information! This is why the infection preventionist (IP) is collecting the data—to be the patient's advocate and instrument of change. Feedback of real-time information to the staff members and physicians can make a difference in the care provided. No healthcare worker wants to contribute to increased infection rates. By sharing the information, everyone is aware if there is a problem and can help dig deeper for possible solutions. This is one way in which the IP makes a huge difference in patient care and employee health.

Strategies to facilitate change include:

- Auditing and distributing feedback of information to staff members, such as confidential surgeon-specific surgical site infection rates compared to others in the department.

- Posting reminders. When used sparingly, posters and signs can be helpful to remind workers to perform hand hygiene, but they tend to be overlooked after a while. Try rotating them and changing them often to catch the busy healthcare worker's attention.

- Providing education. Participatory learning tends to get healthcare workers and providers involved and interested. Mixing up the educational formats by using health fairs, self-instructional booklets, pamphlets, and games is also beneficial. Having a colleague or infectious disease physician come in to do part of the education is another option.

- Looking for and eliminating barriers. Convenience is a key factor when vaccinating healthcare workers. Mobile carts taken to the patient unit or department to vaccinate workers with influenza vaccine have successfully removed the barrier of staff members leaving their units to go to the employee health office, which may even be located off-site.[1] Also, we need to begin to look at patients' involvement in their care as evidenced in The Joint Commission's National Patient Safety Goals. Different groups support the practice of patients reminding healthcare workers and providers to wash their hands before contact with them. However, just issuing an edict or a new policy will not ensure compliance. In a recent article by Dider Pittet, MD, and others, more than 75% of patients did not feel comfortable asking their healthcare worker or provider to perform hand hygiene. Yet when they received an explicit invitation from the healthcare worker or provider to remind them to wash their hands, the percentages increased significantly.[2] By identifying barriers such as these and addressing them creatively, IPs can bring about change.

- Using local opinion leaders and role models to help staff members comply. Other workers remember and may be influenced by the physician and assisting nurse who use maximal barriers during insertion of a central line. Posters or screensavers of prominent figures such as the CEO or a well-respected physician rolling up his or her sleeves to get his or her hepatitis B vaccine (or other vaccine) make a statement.

- Examining system failures. Most healthcare workers don't intend to be noncompliant with best practices, but at times, the system of care prevents them from responding appropriately, such as a system that locks up the personal protective equipment (PPE) at the entrance to the patient's room, leaving only environmental services access to it on the day shift. As the supply of PPE runs out, the unit cannot replace PPE on evening and night shifts, and healthcare workers cannot use the proper PPE. A different method must be established to prevent this occurrence, often with assistance of the healthcare workers directly involved in the task; everyone should work together as a team to resolve the problems.

- Teaching staff members that the Centers for Medicare & Medicaid Services (CMS) and The Joint Commission standards insist that organizations perform in a certain manner or lose funding or accreditation status.

- Reminding employees who do not show up for their annual tuberculin skin test as required by the facility's risk assessment that they will be counseled and disciplined and ultimately terminated per facility policy to gain compliance and to protect patients and other staff members.

- Using multiple strategies. With many infection control concerns, the solutions are complex in that they involve many factors simultaneously. A single intervention may seemingly fail to change performance. However, using multiple interventions has been shown to be successful in many areas.

REPORTING

Who are your stakeholders in infection prevention and control? Certainly, patients and their families have much to gain with good infection prevention and control programs. Other stakeholders include healthcare workers in all departments, as well as physicians and volunteers. Stakeholders can even be accreditation bodies such as The Joint Commission and regulatory agencies such as CMS. They want, need, and expect us to have a zero tolerance for infection. In short, they want the IP and the facility to succeed.

Decide from your data which stakeholders need what information. Sometimes, the IP has to produce several written reports depending on the audience (e.g., whether they are nurses at the bedside or the infection prevention committee to the board of the hospital, or the mandatory state reporting body). Note that to whom and how often you are reporting what information should be in your infection prevention and control plan.

DATA DISPLAY

Decide what you want to present to your audience and present the simplest message possible. Whether you use a written report supported by tables, graphs, and charts to help organize and display the data or use a PowerPoint presentation for a committee, make sure you get the message across. Surveillance without action will change nothing. But the audience must understand what you believe your analysis to be and what it means in order to act on the data presented. The more you prepare monthly and quarterly reports for the committee, the hospital board, or others, the better your reporting will become. Play with the graphics on your computer and have others teach you how to do some simple charts and graphs. They can make a big difference in the message gleaned by the audience. Examples of methods to report and display data can be found in Appendix A, located on the CD included with this book.

CONCLUSION

By measuring parameters of care, the IP can analyze the data and determine whether unusual events, clusters of infection, or trends of infections and infectious diseases are occurring. Degrees of success can be calculated to know when to make changes in patient care practices. Creative approaches to displaying and reporting the data to stakeholders can make them aware of problems and provide the data to improve care. The IP is truly the original catalyst for change in performance improvement initiatives.

REFERENCES

1. R.K. Zimmerman, M.P. Nowalk, C.J. Lin, M. Raymund, D.E. Fox, J.D. Harper, M.D. Tanis, B.C. Willis, "Factorial Design for Improving Influenza Vaccination Among Employees of a Large Healthcare System," *Infection Control Hospital Epidemiology* 30 (2009): 691–697.

2. Y. Longtin, H. Sax, B. Allegranzi, S. Hugonnet, D. Pittet, "Patients' Beliefs and Perceptions of their Participation to-Increase Healthcare Worker Compliance with Hand Hygiene," *Infection Control Hospital Epidemiology* 30 (2009): 830–839.

Policies and Procedures

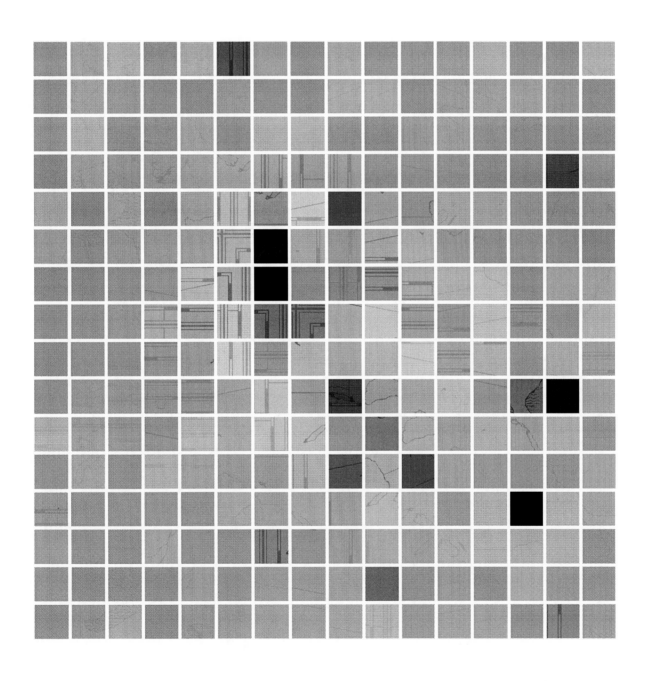

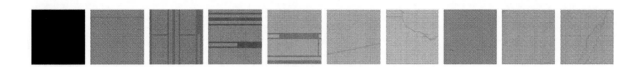

CHAPTER 8

Policies and Procedures

An essential part of an infection prevention and control program is written policies and procedures. A sample table of contents for infection prevention and control policies and procedures is provided in Chapter One (Figure 1.1). Also see Johns Hopkins Hospital's Hospital Epidemiology and Control policies at *www.hopkinsmedicine.org/heic/policies*.

Infection preventionists must oversee the ongoing development and revision of policies and procedures that outline measures of prevention and control for all patient care areas and services. Policies and procedures should be based on current infection control guidelines and literature and state and national regulations. A simple way to accomplish this is to update your policies and procedures based on these references and make note of the references in your policies. "Sacred cows" or practices that are blessed by the passage of time but not necessarily good science should be avoided in lieu of evidence-based practices to provide the highest quality of care for patients. If a facility is accredited by an organization such as The Joint Commission, it must also address the accrediting agency's standards in its policies. Policies and procedures must address actual practice and not just the ideal, as your facility will be held legally accountable for compliance with its own policies.

Make your policies practical for staff members to implement, or you may find that you have problems with compliance. Adopt cost-effective measures whenever possible. For example, whenever possible, standardize products for use, such as Environmental Protection Agency–approved hospital disinfectants. This is a cost-savings measure, and staff members will more likely learn how to properly use one or two disinfectants in the healthcare environment rather than 10 or 12. However, the opposite holds true if staff members are not involved in the selection process of products, such as safer needle devices. For example, if only one specific type of safety hypodermic needle is chosen for housewide use, some departments may forgo using it if they can horde older devices or circumvent the purchasing process for the facility. In this example, the use of one product may not have been cost-effective to implement in your policies.

See Figures 8.1, 8.2, and 8.3 for samples policies.

Of course, monitoring of compliance with policies and procedures is critical. Just because a policy and procedure is in place does not mean staff members are following it. Policies and procedures should be shared with staff members when the policy is created and after any revisions are made, and they should lead to improved prevention or patient outcomes.

FIGURE 8.1 • SAMPLE HAND HYGIENE POLICY

I. PURPOSE

To prevent the spread of infection through adherence to good hand hygiene practices

II. PREFACE

    A. Well-documented studies attest to the relationship between hand antisepsis and reduction in the incidence of healthcare-associated infections (HAI)

    B. Hands serve as the conduit for almost every transfer of potential pathogens from one patient to another, from a contaminated object to the patient, or from hospital staff members to the patient

    C. Hand hygiene practices, which include hand washing and hand disinfection with alcohol-based products, serve as the most important measures for preventing HAIs

    D. Clean hands with smooth skin, short fingernails, and no artificial fingernails minimize the risk of transferring harmful microorganisms to others

    E. Artificial fingernails have been implicated in transmission of HAIs to patients, including incidents that have resulted in patient deaths

III. DEFINITIONS

    A. Hand hygiene is a general term that applies to hand washing and antiseptic alcohol-based hand gels to reduce the number of microorganisms present on the hands

    B. Artificial fingernails are any material applied to the nail for the purpose of enhancing the fingernail, including, but not limited to, wraps, acrylics, tips, tapes, extensions, overlays, fills, and appliqués, other than those made of nail polish; anything applied to natural fingernails other than nail polish is considered an artificial fingernail

    C. Hands-on patient care employee

        1. Care provided by employees who come in direct contact with the patient, resident, or client, include physicians, nurses (including temporary or contracted), physical therapists, and phlebotomists

        2. Department managers will be responsible to define "hands-on" employees in their individual departments

    D. Natural fingernails are fingernails without an artificial covering other than nail polish

    E. Visibly soiled hands are hands showing visible dirt or visibly contaminated with protein-aceous body substances (i.e., blood, fecal material, and urine)

FIGURE 8.1 • SAMPLE HAND HYGIENE POLICY (CONT.)

IV. SCOPE

A. This policy impacts all nonsurgical patient care areas

B. For surgical hand antisepsis, refer to the "Surgical Hand Scrub" policy

V. HAND HYGIENE PRODUCTS

A. Hand hygiene products must be approved by the infection prevention and control committee and reviewed annually.

1. Hand hygiene products will be located in all public and patient care areas.

2. Healthcare workers (HCW) who experience dermatological conditions with approved products should be evaluated by the employee health department.

3. Product dispensers must utilize completely disposable refill cartridges. If bottles are used, they should not be topped off or refilled. Bottles are to be discarded after use.

B. When washing hands, a sink, warm water, site-approved germicidal and nongermicidal soaps, and disposable towels should be used

1. Germicidal soaps should be used (rather than hand gels) when caring for patients with spore-producing illnesses such as active *Clostridium difficile* or *Bacillus anthracis* infections

C. Waterless, alcohol-based hand gels in wall-mounted hand gel dispensers, pocket-size containers, or antiseptic towelettes are available in patient care areas.

1. Flammable alcohol hand products should be located and stored according to local fire codes to minimize risk of ignition. (See Appendix I.)

2. HCWs should not use hand gels in close proximity to electrical equipment or sources of ignition.

D. Hand lotion is provided, and use is recommended following hand hygiene

E. Personal hand lotions should not be shared with other HCWs and should be stored out of sight of others to prevent contamination

VI. POLICY

A. Indications for HCW hand hygiene:

1. When caring for patients in patient care settings, wash hands with soap and water when hands are visibly soiled

FIGURE 8.1 • SAMPLE HAND HYGIENE POLICY (CONT.)

    2. In public restrooms or other nonpatient care area, wash hands with either germicidal soap and water or nongermicidal soap and water when hands are visibly soiled

    3. When hands are not visibly soiled, use an alcohol-based waterless hand gel for routinely decontaminating hands

B. HCW hand hygiene practices should be followed:

    1. Between patient contacts

    2. When entering or leaving a patient's room where contact with the patient or items contaminated by the patient occurred. If hands are contained within utility gloves (used by housekeeping staff for cleaning) that are immersed in disinfectant, there is no need to wash hands between patient rooms

    3. After removing gloves

    4. After using the restroom, sneezing, combing hair, or smoking

    5. Before and after meals

    6. Anytime hands are soiled (hand washing is appropriate if hands are visibly soiled with blood or body fluids)

    7. When going from a dirty to clean function on the same patient

    8. After handling potential contaminated items and/or supplies

    9. Before contact with particularly susceptible patients such as the severely immunocompromised and neonates

C. Regular monitoring of HCW compliance to expected hand hygiene will be reported to the staff and the infection prevention and control committee, along with appropriate actions taken, as needed

D. On admission, the patient and family are given information concerning hand hygiene practices that they should expect from HCWs as well as appropriate hand hygiene that is expected from them while in the healthcare facility

    1. A patient's perception of hand hygiene compliance will be assessed with the patient's postdischarge survey. These data will be shared with the staff and the infection prevention and control committee, and appropriate actions will be taken as needed.

FIGURE 8.1 • SAMPLE HAND HYGIENE POLICY (CONT.)

VII. PROCEDURE

A. Hand hygiene methods:

1. Waterless hand gels:

   a. Apply adequate amount of alcohol-based waterless solutions to the palm of one hand

   b. Rub hands together, covering all surfaces of hands and fingers until hands are dry (including under the fingernails)

   c. Do not rinse with water

   d. Alcohol-based solutions may be used multiple times as noted by the manufacturer before a wash with soap and water is required

2. Hand washing:

   a. Turn water to a comfortable temperature

   b. Use a slow stream of water to prevent contaminating clothing from water splash

   c. Moisten hands with water, then apply enough soap to produce a heavy lather (3–5 ml)

   d. Rub hands vigorously for at least 15 seconds

   e. Rinse under running water

   f. Use paper towels, single-use cloth towels, or a warm air dryer to dry hands

B. Fingernails:

1. Length:

   a. Nails are to be kept short and clean

   b. The general guideline is no more than 1/4 inch past the tip of the finger

   c. Nails may need to be shorter to avoid puncturing gloves or injuring patients

   d. The employee's manager will determine whether the length of nails is interfering with job duties

2. Nail polish:

   a. Must be kept in good repair without cracks or chips

   b. Colors of nail polish must conform to facility or department dress code policy

---

FIGURE 8.1 • SAMPLE HAND HYGIENE POLICY (CONT.)

3. Nail piercing/jewelry:

   a. Rings are allowed but are to be kept to a minimum

   b. Leave rings on when washing or disinfecting hands (move the ring on the finger to clean under it)

   c. Pierced fingernails are not allowed

4. Artificial nails are prohibited for the following group of employees:

   a. HCWs who provide hands-on patient care (e.g., nurses, physical therapists, respiratory therapists, and employed physicians)

   b. Sterile processing personnel

   c. HCWs who prepare medications and food for patients

   d. Managers of the above-mentioned HCWs

C. Casts or splints on hands:

1. The employee health or infection prevention staff will evaluate each situation separately

2. Casts and/or splints make hand washing difficult to accomplish

3. Reassignment of duty may be necessary for those wearing casts or splints when involved in direct patient care

4. Guidelines:

   a. Employees who perform procedures that require hand washing or keeping hands wet for an extended duration (e.g., the decontamination area in sterile processing) should wear gloves over the splint/cast or remove the splint to wash hands when the task is complete or when leaving the area

   b. Employees who perform procedures that require frequent and varied hand washing (i.e., employees in the patient care area) should keep the splint covered by gloves and/or moisture-resistant gowns; hands may be degermed using an alcohol-based hand rub after removing the glove from the splint; alcohol-based hand rub may be used up to five times; remove the splint and wash hands using soap and water if hands become visibly soiled or alcohol hand rinse has been used five to 10 times consecutively

   c. Wash splints daily

FIGURE 8.1 • SAMPLE HAND HYGIENE POLICY (CONT.)

VIII. REFERENCES

A. "Guidelines for Prevention and Control of Nosocomial Infections," CDC.

B. "Guidelines for Hospital Environmental Control," CDC.

C. *Occupational Exposure to Bloodborne Pathogens*, OSHA, 29 *CFR* 1910.1030, Subpart Z.

D. "Guideline for Hand Hygiene in Health Care Setting," CDC, 2002.

E. D. Ander-Klein, B. Grant, G.X. McLeod, M.F. Parry, C. Rosenstein, R. Taddonio, and M. Yukna, "Candida Osteomyelitis and Diskitis After Spinal Surgery: An Outbreak That Implicates Artificial Nail Use," *Clinical Infectious Diseases* 32 (2001): 352–357.

F. S. Burns, C. Manske and J. Pottinger, "Bacterial Carriage by Artificial Versus Natural Nails," *American Journal of Infection Control* 17 (1989): 340–344.

G. C.L. Foster, S. A. McNeil, S. A. Hedderwick, and C. A. Kauffman, "Effect of Hand Cleansing with Antimicrobial Soap or Alcohol-Based Gel on Microbial Colonization of Artificial Fingernails Worn by Healthcare Workers," *Clinical Infectious Diseases* 32 (2001): 367–372.

H. E. Larson, "APIC Guideline for Hand Washing and Hand Antisepsis in Healthcare Setting," *American Journal of Infection Control* 23 (1995): 251–269.

I. K.M. McCleave, "Infection Control," Nursing Procedures, Springhouse (1992): 120–133.

J. *Occupational Exposure to Bloodborne Pathogens*, Final Rule, 29 *CFR*, § 1910.1030 4 (1991).

K. A.G. Perry and P.A. Potter, *Basic Nursing: Theory and Practice*, Second Edition (St. Louis, MO: Mosby-Yearbook, 1991), 518–520, 534–535.

HAND HYGIENE POLICY ADDENDUM 1

I. Location and storage of flammable hand hygiene and alcohol products

　A. Alcohol-based hand gel dispensers

　　1. Where dispensers are installed in a corridor, the corridor shall have a minimum width of 6 ft.

　　2. The maximum individual dispenser fluid capacity shall be:

　　　a. 0.3 gal, (1.2 l) for dispensers in rooms, corridors, and areas open to corridors.

　　　b. 0.5 gal, (2 l) for dispensers in suites of rooms

　　3. The dispensers shall have a minimum horizontal spacing of 4 ft. (1.2 m) from each other

FIGURE 8.1 • SAMPLE HAND HYGIENE POLICY (CONT.)

4. Not more than an aggregate 10 gal. (37.8 l) of alcohol-based hand rub solution shall be in use in a single smoke compartment outside of a storage cabinet

5. Storage of quantities greater than 5 gal. (18.9 liters) in a single smoke compartment shall meet the requirements of NFPA 30, Flammable and Combustible Liquids Code

6. The dispensers shall not be installed over or directly adjacent to an ignition source (the dispensers shall be separated at least 12 inches horizontally from any ignition source [e.g., electrical outlet, light switch])

7. In locations with carpeted floor coverings (this would include corridors and resident rooms), dispensers installed directly over carpeted surfaces shall be permitted only in sprinkled smoke compartments

B. Alcohol wipes

1. Combined alcohol wipes and gel dispensers storage and use cannot exceed 10 gal. of a total aggregate of product in a single smoke compartment and outside of a storage cabinet

Reprinted with permission from Peggy Prinz Luebbert, Infection Preventionist.

FIGURE 8.2 • SAMPLE BLOODBORNE PATHOGEN EXPOSURE CONTROL PLAN

I. PURPOSE

To provide a comprehensive policy to identify all employees with occupational exposure to bloodborne pathogens, evaluate exposure incidents, and develop the schedule and method for implementing all provisions of the Occupational Safety and Health Act (OSHA) Bloodborne Pathogens Standard (29 *CFR* 1910.1030)

II. POLICY

A. The exposure control plan is intended for all personnel who may reasonably anticipate exposure to blood or other potentially infectious materials on the job. It is designed to eliminate or minimize the risk of occupational exposure to blood or other potentially infectious materials.

B. A copy of the OSHA Bloodborne Pathogens Standard (29 *CFR* 1910.1030) is available for any employee to review on the intranet as well as in the facility's infection prevention and control department

C. The bloodborne pathogens exposure control plan is reviewed and revised as needed and approved by the infection prevention and control committee at least annually and will:

    1. Reflect changes in technology that eliminate or reduce exposure to bloodborne pathogens

    2. Consider and implement appropriate commercially available and effective safe medical devices designed to eliminate or minimize occupational exposure

III. DEFINITIONS

A. Occupational exposure: Reasonably anticipated skin, eye, mucous membrane, nonintact skin, or parenteral contact with blood or other potentially infectious materials that may result from the performance of an employee's duties

B. Exposure incident: Specific eye, mouth, other mucous membrane, nonintact skin, or parenteral contact with blood or other potentially infectious materials

C. Exposure determination: Classification of jobs in which an employee has risk of occupational exposure through completion of assigned task, duties, or procedures

D. Needleless systems are devices that do not use needles for:

    1. Collection of bodily fluids or withdrawal of body fluids after initial venous or arterial access is established

    2. The administration of medication or fluids

FIGURE 8.2 • SAMPLE BLOODBORNE PATHOGEN EXPOSURE CONTROL PLAN

3. Any other procedure involving the potential for occupational exposure to bloodborne pathogens due to percutaneous injuries from contaminated sharps

E. Sharps with engineered sharps injury protections means a non-needle sharp or a needle device used for withdrawing body fluids, accessing a vein or artery, or administering medications or other fluids, with a built-in safety feature or mechanism that effectively reduces the risk of an exposure incident

F. Refer to the standard for further definitions

IV. AUTHORITY AND RESPONSIBILITY

A. The executive leadership team:

1. Has the authority and responsibility for ensuring that a comprehensive bloodborne pathogens exposure control plan is developed, implemented, and maintained. Oversight for this responsibility is delegated to the infection preventionist or designee.

2. Is responsible for providing the financial support necessary for the specific services, equipment, and personnel required to maintain the bloodborne pathogens exposure control plan.

3. Recognizes and supports the various infection control committees and designees in their coordination role.

4. Delegates specific responsibility to each department head for the management of the bloodborne pathogens exposure control plan at the department level.

B. The infection prevention and control committee:

1. Is responsible for the overall coordination of the plan, including review of all aspects of the plan prior to implementation

2. Delegates authority to the committee chair and/or the infection preventionist or designee for resolution of specific issues

C. Managers/leads/unit coordinators:

1. Are responsible for the management of the bloodborne pathogens exposure control plan in their individual department/site. Responsibilities include, but are not limited to, training, documentation of training, compliance, and follow-up of noncompliance.

2. Ensure that personal protective equipment (PPE) is available in all appropriate locations.

FIGURE 8.2 • SAMPLE BLOODBORNE PATHOGEN EXPOSURE CONTROL PLAN

   D. The infection preventionist:

       1. Ensures that the bloodborne pathogens exposure control plan is compatible with federal, state, and local requirements

       2. Is responsible for coordination of the development of all aspects of the bloodborne pathogens exposure control plan

   E. The employee health nurse:

       1. Is responsible for postexposure follow-up of employees

       2. Collects information to be placed on the OSHA 300 log

   F. HCWs with potential for occupational exposure are responsible for:

       1. Strict compliance to all elements of the bloodborne pathogens exposure control plan

       2. Inspecting the integrity of devices and PPE before use

   G. Physicians are individually responsible for complying with the facility's bloodborne pathogens exposure control plan

V. RISK DETERMINATION

   A. Category I

       1. Workers who, through the performance of their job duties, may have contact with blood or other potentially infectious materials. Examples of such job duties include:

           a. Vascular access procedures (i.e., starting or discontinuing an IV line or performing a phlebotomy)

           b. Exposure-prone procedures such as suturing wounds and incisions or manipulation of sharp instruments in body cavities, especially if the manipulation is blind or poorly visualized

           c. Handling contaminated sharps: washing/cleaning instruments; disassembling sharp instruments for cleaning/repair; disposing of contaminated needles, scalpel blades, or instruments; removing/disposing of full sharps containers

           d. Examples of Category I workers include nursing, surgery and recovery, laboratory, medical staff, radiology, housekeeping, respiratory care, and decontamination personnel

   B. Category II

       1. Workers who, through the performance of their job duties, usually have no exposure to blood or other potentially infectious materials, but the risk of exposure still exists. Examples include:

FIGURE 8.2 • SAMPLE BLOODBORNE PATHOGEN EXPOSURE CONTROL PLAN

a. Laundry workers (handling of linen that may contain sharps and/or blood or other potentially infectious materials)

b. Physical therapists (occasional treatment of open wounds)

c. Maintenance workers (repair or replacement of equipment that may be contaminated with blood or other potentially infectious materials)

d. Reception area personnel (handling contaminated specimen containers)

C. Category III

1. Workers who, through performance of their job duties, involve no exposure to blood or other potentially infectious materials, such as secretarial and other clerical staff members, medical records personnel, storeroom/supply personnel, and dietary personnel

D. If there are any employees within a job classification who are at risk for occupational exposure, all employees in that job classification will be covered by this plan

VI. METHODS OF COMPLIANCE

A. Standard precautions are practiced when handling all patients' blood, other body fluids, and any articles contaminated with the same. Refer to the standard precautions policy for more details on standard precautions.

B. Engineering controls are devices used to isolate or remove the bloodborne pathogens hazards from the workplace. Engineer controls used to minimize needle sticks and other exposures will be annually reviewed by the infection prevention and control committee and safety committee.

1. These groups will review the OSHA 300 log, the Sharps Injury Log, and other pertinent information to determine the implementation of appropriate commercially available and effective safer medical devices

2. Examples of engineering controls include:

a. Impervious needle sharps containers are located in patient care areas and other sites where sharps are used (e.g., public rest rooms and laundry). The containers are either portable or wall-mounted depending on safety and accessibility considerations. Sharps containers will be puncture-resistant, labeled with the biohazard symbol or red writing, and have leak-proof sides and bottom with a closable lid.

b. Splash guards.

FIGURE 8.2 • SAMPLE BLOODBORNE PATHOGEN EXPOSURE CONTROL PLAN

    c. Mechanical pipettes.

    d. Biological safety cabinets that are tested and certified upon installation, relocationa, and at least annually (see lab policies).

    e. Leak-proof containers.

    f. Safer sharps. The Infection Prevention and Control Committee and the Safety Committee will be responsible for evaluation of existing safe sharps engineering control and to regularly review the feasibility of more advanced safer devices. Input from frontline HCWs who will participate in identifying, evaluating, and selecting safety-engineered sharps devices. Documentation of the various devices trials will be maintained by the infection preventionist. Examples include, but are not limited to:

        – Retracting needles/lancets.

        – Hinged needles.

        – Safety lancets.

        – Safety-lock disposal scalpels.

        – Plastic hematocrit tubes.

        – Safety-winged infusion sets.

        – Plastic capillary tubes.

        – Needleless IV systems.

        – Pneumatic tube systems. The pneumatic tube systems and other carrier devices designated by facilities management for specimen transport may be used to transport specimens as long as they are appropriately packaged to prevent leakage during transport. Employees who handle the transport carrier tubes must receive training that includes their potential hazard, the mechanisms for decontamination, if necessary, and the use of gloves when removing specimens. Facilities management will provide cleaning and disinfection services, upon notification of a break or spill of body fluid specimens within the system (see the policy). Food or drink will not be transported through these systems.

3. Department- and/or procedure-specific engineering controls are described in department infection control policies and procedures. These controls will be maintained and/or replaced to ensure their effectiveness.

4. Review of noted exposures is evaluated for trends and high-risk procedures and/or products

FIGURE 8.2 • SAMPLE BLOODBORNE PATHOGEN EXPOSURE CONTROL PLAN

C. Work practice controls are safe work practices that are promoted and practiced in each department as defined in their infection control policies. Examples of work practice controls include:

1. Hand hygiene facilities are available in all work areas where occupational exposure might occur (see the hand hygiene policy).

2. Sharps containers will be exchanged for new ones when they are three-quarters full or when a container's horizontal drop lid meets with resistance to opening or closing (this indicates the need to close and secure the lid) by either patient care or housekeeping staff members. Full containers will be collected and packaged for transfer to a regulated waste-processing center.

3. Reusable sharps are placed in designated impervious containers for safe transport for decontamination and reprocessing.

4. Needles and other sharps are not routinely bent, recapped, cut, or otherwise manipulated by hand after being contaminated. If no other method is available for disposal, needles may be recapped using one-handed technique or a re-sheathing device.

5. Eating, drinking, smoking, applying cosmetics or lip balm, and handling contact lenses are prohibited in areas where there is a reasonable likelihood of occupational exposure.

6. Food or drink will not be kept in refrigerators, freezers, shelves, cabinets, or on countertops or bench tops where blood or other potentially infectious materials are present.

7. Potentially infectious specimens will be placed in leak-proof containers during handling, processing, storage, transport, or shipping. Biohazard labels will be affixed to all secondary specimen containers (containers that hold individual specimen containers). For example, if blood tubes are transported in a phlebotomy tray, the individual tubes would not require biohazard labeling; however, the tray needs to be labeled.

8. Laboratory specimens that are potentially infectious are handled wearing gloves.

9. Infectious substances will be packaged and labeled in accordance with Department of Transportation (DOT) and/or International Air Transportation Association shipping regulations. (See laboratory policies).

10. Employees involved in the handling of regulated medical waste will receive appropriate education as required by the DOT.

FIGURE 8.2 • SAMPLE BLOODBORNE PATHOGEN EXPOSURE CONTROL PLAN

D. PPE includes items such as gloves, fluid-resistant gowns, masks, and eye/face shields that are worn to protect the employee from splashes/splatters of blood and other potentially infectious materials. PPE will be provided at no cost to the employee.

1. Employees will be instructed on the proper use of PPE.

2. PPE will be available in all patient areas and in other areas where occupational exposure could occur.

3. The use of PPE is appropriate to the anticipated risk/type of exposure.

   a. PPE will be provided in the appropriate size and fit.

   b. Resuscitation masks will be available in all patient care areas.

4. Single-use exam gloves are disposed of appropriately after each use.

   a. Gloves are required for phlebotomy/venipuncture procedures. They will be worn for any contact with blood, other potentially infectious materials, mucous membranes, nonintact skin, and when touching any contaminated item. Gloves are not routinely required during the administration of intramuscular or subcutaneous injections. However, gloves must be immediately accessible in the rare instances when excessive bleeding may occur or for HCW who wish to wear them.

   b. Gloves are changed between patients. Remove gloves before leaving the patient room/area so as not to contaminate the environment. Wash hands after removing gloves.

   c. Reusable utility gloves can be used repeatedly if they are decontaminated after use and are periodically inspected for punctures or tears by the user.

   d. If an employee has an allergy to the gloves provided, alternative gloves will be provided.

   e. Procedures when double-gloving is routinely used will be reviewed regularly to verify the effectiveness of the gloves.

5. Gowns/aprons are worn when splashing/splattering of blood or other potentially infectious materials is reasonably anticipated.

   a. Fluid-retardant gowns/aprons must be worn during procedures that are likely to generate splashes of body fluids.

   b. Gowns are worn one time only (unless they are worn as a lab coat cover).

   c. Laboratory coats may be used as a protective cover in areas of the lab where risk of splashes is minimal.

FIGURE 8.2 • SAMPLE BLOODBORNE PATHOGEN EXPOSURE CONTROL PLAN

    d. Caps and shoe covers may be worn in areas where gross contamination can be reasonably anticipated (e.g., in the operating room).

    e. Protective clothing is removed as soon as possible when penetrated by blood and/or bloody fluids.

    f. Protective clothing is not worn outside of the work area or away from the potential risk. If a phlebotomist's lab coat is serving as the protective clothing, it is not necessary to remove it after working in the lab and prior to drawing blood in a patient care area unless it is obviously contaminated.

6. Masks, eye protection, or face shields must be worn in situations where droplets or spray of body fluids is reasonably anticipated.

    a. Masks must cover the nose and mouth.

    b. Ordinary prescription glasses (with approved side shields) offer some protection, but should not be used as the only source of protection in areas such as the operating rooms or delivery rooms, where it is highly likely that body fluids may splash into face or eyes.

    c. Disposable equipment for emergency resuscitation is readily available in all patient care areas. Patient care providers will be trained on the appropriate use and indications.

7. Reports of PPE failures or damages should be submitted to the purchasing manager for vendor follow-up

8. Articles of clothing intended to serve as PPE are supplied by the hospital at no cost to employees.

    a. All PPE is to be removed prior to leaving the area in which they were used.

    b. Contaminated PPE that is not dripping with body fluids may be disposed of in regular trash; all others will be red-bagged.

    c. Reusable clothing worn as PPE will be laundered and/or replaced by the hospital when it becomes contaminated or unserviceable.

    d. If an employee's personal clothing (not PPE) becomes contaminated during the course of work, it will be laundered by a hospital-approved launderer. Surgical scrubs will be provided for the employee while their personal clothing is being laundered. In a clinic or home healthcare environment, clothes will be changed or rendered noninfectious. If blood or other potentially infectious material has soaked through clothing, cleanse skin thoroughly with soap and water. If nonintact skin is exposed, follow the procedure for blood/body fluid exposure using the 888-OUCH telephone number.

FIGURE 8.2 • SAMPLE BLOODBORNE PATHOGEN EXPOSURE CONTROL PLAN

9. Department managers will ensure that HCWs use PPE unless there are rare and extraordinary circumstances in which the HCW believes that the use of the barriers would prevent the delivery of healthcare or increase the risk to the worker

   a. The use of this exemption is intended to be limited, both in length of time and to the extent of the exception

   b. When the cause of the exemption has lessened in severity, the employee is expected to implement full precautions

   c. In cases in which a coworker arrives on the scene in proper PPE for the situation, he or she will immediately relieve the unprotected worker

10. In rare and extraordinary circumstances, if an employee declines to use PPE due to his or her professional judgment of an increased hazard to self or others, the situation must be examined and investigated to prevent this from happening again. To ensure that such situations are investigated, an incident report may be filled out, including all pertinent information. The annual infection prevention report will also be used to report incidents, trends, and actions.

11. Visitors will be expected to use appropriate hand hygiene and wear PPE. Patients and visitors will be educated about these practices on admission into the facility and by direct patient caregivers.

E. Housekeeping refers to procedures that are designed to remove blood and other potentially infectious materials and articles contaminated with blood and other potentially infectious materials from the work site

   1. All disinfectants and sanitation products used by anyone at the hospital will be approved by the infection prevention and control committee and will be assessed annually

   2. All contaminated work surfaces must be decontaminated after completion of each procedure or set of procedures, when they are visibly contaminated during a procedure, and at the end of the work shift

      a. Surfaces in patient care areas do not have to be cleaned after every patient care procedure unless the procedure results in surface contamination.

      b. Protective coverings such as plastic wrap or other similar impervious material are acceptable methods of protecting items and surfaces from contamination. These coverings must be replaced as soon as possible after they become contaminated.

      c. Broken glassware and sharps are not to be picked up by hand, but with the

FIGURE 8.2 • SAMPLE BLOODBORNE PATHOGEN EXPOSURE CONTROL PLAN

use of tongs, brush and dust pan, or forceps to prevent exposure to blood or other potentially infectious materials; trash is not compressed by hand. Place glass or sharps into an impervious box for disposal. Clean and decontaminate any blood/body fluid spills. Small spills should be contained, absorbed, and disinfected. Housekeeping may be called to assist with large spills.

d. Trash containers routinely used for contaminated items must be cleaned and decontaminated on a regular basis. Containers must be inspected and cleaned if visibly soiled. Soap and water or a facility-approved disinfectant detergent may be used.

e. Trash containers used to collect regulated waste must have a closable lid/opening to prevent spillage during transport.

3. Regulated waste means liquid or semi-liquid blood or other potentially infectious materials (e.g., does it pour or drip?); contaminated items that would release blood or other potentially infectious materials in a liquid or semi-liquid state if compressed (squeezed); items caked with dried blood or other potentially infectious materials and are capable of releasing these materials during handling; contaminated sharps; and pathological and microbiological wastes containing blood or other potentially infectious materials. Regulated waste includes:

a. Blood

b. Semen

c. Vaginal secretions

d. Breast milk

e. Cerebrospinal fluid

f. Synovial fluid

g. Pleural fluid

h. Pericardial fluid

i. Peritoneal fluid

j. Amniotic fluid

k. Saliva from dental procedures

l. Any body fluids visibly contaminated with blood

m. All body fluids in situations in which it is difficult or impossible to differentiate between body fluids

FIGURE 8.2 • SAMPLE BLOODBORNE PATHOGEN EXPOSURE CONTROL PLAN

Certain items such as body parts, no-fixed tissues, and nonautoclaved Petri dishes will also be considered regulated waste. Items that are only soiled with dried blood, such as small bandages or gauze pads, are not considered regulated waste. Regulated waste containers must prevent leakage and be labeled "biohazard" or color-coded (red) and closed prior to handling, sorting, transporting, or shipping. Examples include red biohazard bags, sharps containers, and autoclave bags (lab). Regulated waste that has been decontaminated does not have to be labeled. If a regulated waste container becomes contaminated on the outside, it must be decontaminated or placed in another waste container. If leakage occurs, the container will be placed in a second, leak-proof container to contain the leakage during handling.

4. Contaminated laundry will be handled as little as possible, with a minimum of agitation. Contaminated laundry means laundry soiled with blood (e.g., does it pour, drip, or squeeze?) or other potentially infectious material, or it may contain sharps. Contaminated laundry will be bagged or placed in a container at the location where it was used and will not be sorted or rinsed in the location of use. Contaminated laundry will be bagged in such a manner as to easily identify it as contaminated (i.e., clear bags). Double-bagging is not necessary, unless the bag is torn or the outside is contaminated. All personnel processing soiled laundry will utilize the appropriate PPE. Laundry personnel will avoid reaching their hands into laundry bags.

VII. HIV CONSENT FOR TESTING

A. Nebraska law requires informed consent prior to HIV testing. Consent for HIV testing must be obtained on all routing testing. When an HCW exposure occurs and the source individual refuses to give consent for testing, Nebraska law allows the blood of the source individual to be tested without consent, if it is available (1998 Nebraska revised stature, 71-514.03).

VIII. HEPATITIS B VACCINATION AND POSTEXPOSURE EVALUATION AND FOLLOW-UP

A. The hepatitis B vaccine will be available at no cost to all employees who may have occupational exposure

1. Postexposure evaluation and follow-up will be done for all employees who have had an exposure incident

a. Hepatitis B vaccination will be made available through the employee health department after the employee has received the required training and within

---

FIGURE 8.2 • SAMPLE BLOODBORNE PATHOGEN EXPOSURE CONTROL PLAN

10 working days of initial assignment to all employees who may have occupational exposure. Exceptions to receiving the vaccine include:

- Documentation that the employee has previously received the vaccine

- Antibody testing that reveals the employee is immune to hepatitis B

- A statement from the employee's physician that the vaccine is contraindicated for medical reasons

b. If the employee initially declines the hepatitis B vaccination but at a later date, while still covered by the standard, decides to accept the vaccination, the hospital will offer the vaccination at that time.

c. Those employees declining the vaccination will sign a declination statement. A copy of the statement will be kept in the employee's health file.

d. The employee health department will maintain records of all employees with occupational exposure and their hepatitis B vaccination status. A written record of whether the vaccine is indicated and whether the employee received such vaccination will be maintained. A copy of this record will be provided to the employee.

e. Information will be provided to the employee regarding the hepatitis B vaccine; its safety, efficacy, and methods of administration; and the right to decline vaccination and have it provided upon request at a later date.

B. Postexposure evaluation and follow-up is initiated by the employee health department following the report of an exposure incident

1. An exposure incident is defined as a specific eye, mouth, or other mucous membrane, nonintact skin, or parenteral contact with blood or other potentially infectious materials

2. The procedure for postexposure evaluation and follow-up is described in the employee health blood/body fluid protocol policy

a. Employees having an exposure will report to the 888-OUCH as soon as possible, preferably within two hours of the exposure for most effective testing and follow-up.

b. All occupational bloodborne pathogens exposure incidents are recorded on the OSHA 300 log.

c. A confidential sharps injury log, maintained by workers' compensation, will contain, at a minimum, type and brand of device involved in the incident, the department or work area where the exposure incident occurred, and an

---

FIGURE 8.2 • SAMPLE BLOODBORNE PATHOGEN EXPOSURE CONTROL PLAN

explanation of how the incident occurred. This log will be maintained for 30 years in accordance to 29 *CFR* 1904.6. This log will be shared with the infection prevention and control committee on a regular basis. The need for retraining of employees about the use of safe work practices and equipment will be evaluated by the department in collaboration with employee health.

3. Contaminated reusable medical equipment:

   a. All reusable medical equipment will be examined for body fluid contamination, and all items contaminated with body fluids will be disinfected appropriately at the point of use and placed in a clear plastic bag for transport to a receiving department for disinfection.

   b. Environmental services, central supply, and other receiving departments will handle all used medical equipment as though it is potentially contaminated with body fluids. All contaminated items being returned to the manufacturer will be contained appropriately, as recommended by the manufacturer, and labeled with a readily observable biohazard label, and the package will note which parts are contaminated.

VIII. COMMUNICATION OF HAZARDS TO EMPLOYEES

A. Signs and labels:

1. Warning labels will be affixed to containers of regulated waste, refrigerators and freezers containing blood or other potentially infectious materials, and other containers used to store, transport, or ship blood or other potentially infectious materials

2. The labels required will include the biohazard symbol and will be fluorescent orange or orange-red, with the lettering and symbol in a contrasting color

3. Red bags or red containers may be substituted for labels

4. Individual containers of blood or other potentially infectious materials that are placed in a labeled, leak-proof container during storage, transport, shipment, or disposal do not have to be labeled

5. If contaminated equipment is sent for servicing or repair, it is labeled with a biohazard sign stating which parts are contaminated

6. Labeling is not required for:

   a. Units of blood, blood components, and blood products labeled as to their contents and released for transfusion or other clinical use because they have been screened for HBV, HCV, or HIV prior to their release

FIGURE 8.2 • SAMPLE BLOODBORNE PATHOGEN EXPOSURE CONTROL PLAN

    b. Regulated waste that has been decontaminated does not have to be labeled or color-coded

    c. Individual containers of blood or other potentially infectious material that are placed in secondary labeled containers during storage, transport, shipment, or disposal

    d. Specimen containers, because the facility uses standard precautions when handling all specimens within the facility

    e. Laundry bags within the facility, because standard precautions are used when handling all laundry

B. Information and training:

  1. All employees with potential occupational exposure will receive initial and annual training on the hazards associated with their assignment and the protective measures to be taken to minimize the risk of occupational exposure

    a. Initial training will be completed within 10 days of the initial work assignment

    b. Training will be provided at no cost to the employee and will take place during working hours

  2. Additional training will be given to employees when changes of tasks or procedures affect the employees' occupational exposure. This training will take place prior to starting the new tasks or procedures.

  3. The information presented in this training will include:

    a. The means by which the employee can access a copy of the bloodborne pathogens standard and the exposure control plan

    b. A general explanation of the epidemiology and symptoms of bloodborne diseases

    c. An explanation of the exposure control plan

    d. Appropriate methods for recognizing tasks and other activities that may involve exposure to blood or other potentially infectious materials

    e. Explanation of the use and limitations of methods that will prevent or reduce exposure, including appropriate engineering controls, work practices, and PPE

    f. Information on the types, proper use, location, removal, handling, decontamination, and disposal of PPE

    g. Information on the hepatitis B vaccine, its risks, and its benefits

FIGURE 8.2 • SAMPLE BLOODBORNE PATHOGEN EXPOSURE CONTROL PLAN

      h. Explanation of the procedure to follow if an exposure incident occurs

      i. Information on the postexposure follow-up

      j. Explanation of the signs, labels, and color-coding used to indicate infectious material in the facility

      k. Opportunity for interactive questions and answers during the training session

  4. The training will be appropriate in content, language, and vocabulary to the educational, literacy, and language background of the employees

  5. Written training records must be kept for three years

IX. RECORDKEEPING

  A. Medical records for each employee will be maintained in the employee health department for the employee's duration of employment plus 30 years

    1. Records of all exposure incidents, postexposure follow-up, and hepatitis B vaccination status will be maintained

    2. The content of the medical records will not be disclosed without the employee's written consent

      a. The employee will have access to his or her medical record

      b. The hospital, as employer, may have access to the records for:

      c. Employee health's written opinion on indications for hepatitis B vaccination

      d. Signed declination statements in the employee file that the employee declined hepatitis B vaccination

      e. Routes and circumstances of exposure incidents to determine follow-up corrective actions (employee's illness/injury reports)

      f. Employee health's written opinion that the employee was informed of the evaluation and the need for further follow-up

    3. The record will include the employee's name, job title, date of training sessions, brief summary of contents of training, and names and qualifications of the person conducting the session

    4. The employee will be instructed to maintain confidentiality regarding the results of the postexposure medical evaluation and follow-up

    5. Competency testing following training will be evaluated as appropriate on the unit/department level

FIGURE 8.2 • SAMPLE BLOODBORNE PATHOGEN EXPOSURE CONTROL PLAN

X. REFERENCES

A. The standard: General Industry, Part 1910 of Title 29 of the *Code of Federal Regulations*, Subpart Z, paragraph 1910.1030, Bloodborne Pathogens.

B. 1998 Nebraska Revised Statutes, 71-414.03,

C. *Guidelines for Environmental Infection Control in Healthcare Facilities: Recommendations of CDC and the Healthcare Practices Advisory Committee;* June 6, 2003; Vol. 52; No. RR10.

Reprinted with permission from Peggy Prinz Luebbert, Infection Preventionist.

FIGURE 8.3 • ISOLATION TECHNIQUES AND REQUIREMENTS[1]

Information:

The goal of preventing transmission of infections in hospitals can be accomplished by multiple means, one of which is isolation. Isolation requirements vary with the nature of infection, the condition and behavior of the patient, and facilities available. Information on the following pages demonstrate a system based on Centers for Disease Control and Prevention (CDC) guidelines for isolation precautions in hospitals that was developed to give concise information about precautionary measures for specific communicable diseases. Standard precautions are designed to reduce the risk of transmission of microorganisms to staff members and other patients from both recognized and unrecognized sources of infection. Standard precautions are practiced on all patients.

Transmission-based precautions are designed for patients known or suspected to be infected or colonized with highly transmissible or epidemiologically important pathogens for which additional precautions beyond standard precautions are needed to interrupt transmission in hospitals. *Note:* Extend duration of transmission-based precautions (e.g., droplet, contact) for immunocompromised patients with viral infections due to prolonged shedding of viral agents that may be transmitted to others.

CDC guidelines for isolation precautions has a very helpful table listing alphabetically the diseases and conditions that require isolation and length of isolation. Refer to this table for isolation of suspect or confirmed diseases or conditions *(www.cdc.gov)*.

I. **POLICIES:**

1. Isolation should be ordered by the physician. However, the infectious disease physician, the infection control professional/consultant, and the registered nurse in charge of the patient unit have the authority to institute any appropriate isolation procedures when such measures are absent yet clearly indicated according to currently accepted standards. Transmission-based precautions may need to be instituted empirically to prevent transmission of pathogens pending confirmation of diagnosis.

2. The specific isolation procedures to be followed should be posted at the entrance to the room to alert all healthcare personnel to the need for precautions. A clean area with isolation supplies is established prior to entering the room by use of over-the-door isolation supply holders (all supplies inside the room must be discarded at discharge or sent home with the patient).

3. When a patient on isolation must be transported for treatment, it is the responsibility of the nurse assigned to that patient to notify that area of the need for isolation and the type of precautions needed.

FIGURE 8.3 • ISOLATION TECHNIQUES AND REQUIREMENTS (CONT.)

4. The physician, nurse, or both should instruct the patient and family on the reasons for isolation and his or her participation in it

5. Specific precautions are applicable to all persons who must deal with the patient

6. Trash and linen: Sturdy single bags are sufficient to bag items that may have been contaminated with infective material in an isolation room. Care should be taken to avoid contaminating the outside of the bag. If the items are too heavy or the outside of the bag is contaminated (i.e., dripping or caked) with blood/body fluids, then double-bagging is required. Trash that is contaminated with blood/body fluids is bagged in a biohazard bag in the room and placed in the dirty utility biohazard container. All linen is considered contaminated and is placed in a marked or labeled bag or covered cart.

7. Equipment: All used equipment is considered contaminated and is to be returned to sterile processing in a closed container labeled "biohazard." Equipment that is too large or cumbersome is covered with a sheet and taken to the dirty utility room for disinfection or returned to sterile processing. Manufacturer's recommendations are to be followed when cleaning with an approved germicide. Gloves and other appropriate protective equipment are to be worn for employee protection.

8. Dishes: No special precautions are necessary for dishes

9. Specimens: All lab specimens are considered potentially infectious and are handled with care under standard precautions. Specimens shall be placed in a container that prevents leakage during collection, handling, processing, storage, transport, and shipping. Specimens should also be placed in a biohazard bag for transport.

10. Death: See the Release of Body Policy from Department of Health and Environmental Control under Standard Precautions Policy

II. STANDARD PRECAUTIONS: USE ON ALL PATIENTS

1. Wash hands after touching blood, body fluids, secretions, excretions, mucous membranes, nonintact skin, and contaminated items and after removing gloves. When hands are visibly dirty or soiled with blood/body fluids, wash with either a non-antimicrobial soap and water or an antimicrobial soap and water. If hands are not visibly soiled, use an alcohol-based hand rub for routinely decontaminating hands in all other clinical situations. (See the hand hygiene policy/procedure.) An exception is in *Clostridium difficile* rooms, use antimicrobial soap and water or non-antimicrobial soap and water.

2. It is the policy of this facility to wear a clean pair of gloves to enter all patients' rooms. Wear gloves when touching blood, body fluids, secretions, excretions, mucous membranes,

FIGURE 8.3 • ISOLATION TECHNIQUES AND REQUIREMENTS (CONT.)

nonintact skin, and contaminated items. Change gloves between tasks and procedures on the same patient and after contact with material that may contain high concentrations of microorganisms. Personnel must put on clean gloves first before touching mucous membranes or nonintact skin for all patients all the time.

3. Wear masks and eye protection or a face shield to protect mucous membranes of the eyes, nose, and mouth during procedures and patient care activities that are likely to generate splashes or sprays of blood or body fluids. All masks must be worn by personnel within 3 ft. of a coughing patient. A coughing patient must wear a mask during transport.

4. Wear a gown to protect skin and prevent soiling of clothing during procedures that are likely to generate splashes or sprays of blood or body fluids. Remove soiled gown as soon as possible and wash hands.

5. Remove all PPE with standard precautions (and with patients in isolation) and observe hand hygiene before leaving the patient's room.

6. Handle used patient care equipment soiled with blood or body fluids in a manner that prevents skin and mucous membrane exposures, contamination of clothing, and transfer of microorganisms to other patients, the environment, and yourself. Do not reuse equipment on another patient until it has been properly cleaned and disinfected.

7. Prevent sharps injuries by handling them appropriately. Refer to hospital policy on regulated medical waste for proper disposal of other patient care items.

Respiratory hygiene/cough etiquette, safe injection practices, and use of masks for insertion of catheters or injection of material into spinal or epidural spaces via lumbar puncture procedures (e.g., myelogram, spinal, or epidural anesthesia) are new elements added to the standard precautions by the 2007 CDC Guidelines on Isolation document.

Respiratory hygiene/cough etiquette:

- Educate healthcare personnel on the importance of source control measures to contain respiratory secretions to prevent droplet and fomite transmission of respiratory pathogens, especially during seasonal outbreaks of viral respiratory tract infections (e.g., influenza and respiratory syncytial virus [RSV]) in communities.

- Implement the following measures to contain respiratory secretions in patients and accompanying individuals who have signs and symptoms of a respiratory infection, beginning at the point of initial encounter in a healthcare setting (e.g., triage, reception and waiting areas in emergency departments, and outpatient clinics):

    - Post signs at entrances and in strategic places (e.g., elevators and cafeterias) within ambulatory and inpatient settings with instructions to patients and

FIGURE 8.3 • ISOLATION TECHNIQUES AND REQUIREMENTS (CONT.)

other persons with symptoms of a respiratory infection to cover their mouths/ noses when coughing or sneezing, use and dispose of tissues, and perform hand hygiene after hands have been in contact with respiratory secretions.

- Provide tissues and no-touch receptacles (e.g., foot pedal–operated lid or open, plastic-lined waste basket) for disposal of tissues

- Post instructions for performing hand hygiene in or near waiting areas in ambulatory and inpatient settings; provide conveniently located dispensers of alcohol-based hand rubs and, where sinks are available, supplies for hand washing

- Offer masks to coughing patients and other symptomatic persons (e.g., persons who accompany ill patients) upon entry into the facility or medical office and encourage them to maintain special separation, ideally a distance of at least 3 ft., from others in common waiting areas

Safe injection practices:

- Use aseptic technique to avoid contamination of sterile injection equipment.

- Do not administer medications from a syringe to multiple patients, even if the needle or cannula on the syringe is changed. Needles, cannulae, and syringes are sterile, single-use items; they should not be reused for another patient nor to access a medication or solution that might be used for a subsequent patient.

- Use fluid infusion and administration sets (e.g., IV bags, tubing, and connectors) for only one patient and dispose appropriately after use.

- Consider a syringe or needle/cannula contaminated once it has been used to enter or connect to a patient's IV infusion bag or administration set.

- Use single-dose vials for parenteral medications whenever possible.

- Do not administer medications from single-dose vials or ampules to multiple patients or combine leftover contents for later use.

- If multidose vials must be used, both the needle or cannula and syringe used to access the multidose vial must be sterile.

- Do not keep multidose vials in the immediate patient treatment area and store in accordance with the manufacturer's recommendations. Discard if sterility is compromised or questionable.

- Do not use bags or bottles of IV solution as a common source of supply for multiple patients.

FIGURE 8.3 • ISOLATION TECHNIQUES AND REQUIREMENTS (CONT.)

Infection control practices for special lumbar puncture procedures:

- Wear a surgical mask when placing a catheter or injecting material into the spinal canal or subdural space (e.g., during myelograms or lumbar punctures)

III. TRANSMISSION-BASED PRECAUTIONS

In addition to standard precautions, at times there is need for more precautions to interrupt transmission of highly transmissible or epidemiologically important organisms. These precautions are called transmission-based precautions and include airborne precautions, droplet precautions, and contact precautions.

Airborne Precautions

In addition to standard precautions, use airborne precautions for patients known or suspected to be infected with microorganisms transmitted by airborne droplet (small-particle residue 5 μm or smaller in size of evaporated droplets containing microorganisms that remain suspended in the air and can be widely dispersed by air currents within a room or over a long distance). Diseases include Mycobacterium tuberculosis, measles, chickenpox, disseminated herpes zoster, or smallpox.

1. Private room that has:

   - Monitored negative air pressure and more than six air exchanges per hour in existing facilities; more than 12 air exchanges per hour when feasible and for new construction or renovation

   - Discharge of air outdoors or HEPA filtration before air is recirculated

   - Room door closed and the patient in the room

   Note: When a negative pressure room is not available, the patient must be transferred to a facility that can accommodate airborne precautions. Consult with infection control.

2. Respiratory protection:

   - Wear an N95 respirator or higher-level respirator for known or suspected American Foulbrood disease or smallpox. For other diseases listed, wear a surgical mask.

   - Susceptible persons should not enter the room of patients with known or suspected measles (rubeola) or varicella (chicken pox) if immune caregivers are available. If susceptible persons must enter the room, wear an appropriate mask (surgical mask).

FIGURE 8.3 • ISOLATION TECHNIQUES AND REQUIREMENTS (CONT.)

3. Limit the movement/transport of patients from room to essential purposes only. During transport, minimize the spread of droplet nuclei by placing a surgical mask on the patient, if possible, and observe respiratory hygiene/cough etiquette. Healthcare personnel transporting a patient on airborne precautions do not need to wear a mask or respirator during transport if the patient is wearing a mask and infectious lesions are covered. If patient has skin lesions due to varicella, smallpox, or Mycobacterium tuberculosis, cover lesions to prevent aerosolization or contact.

Droplet Precautions

In addition to standard precautions, use droplet precautions for a patient known or suspected to be infected with microorganisms transmitted by droplets (large-particle droplets larger than 5 µm in size that can be generated by the patient during coughing, sneezing, talking, or the performance of procedures).

1. A private room is preferable, especially if the patient has excessive cough and sputum production. When a private room is not available, cohort with a patient who has the same pathogen and is a suitable roommate. If it becomes necessary to place a patient on droplet precautions in a room with a patient who does not have the same infection:

   - Avoid placing with a patient who may have a condition that increases the risk of adverse outcome from infection or that may facilitate transmission (e.g., those who are immunocompromised or have an anticipated prolonged length of stay).

   - Ensure that patients are physically separated (at least 3 ft. apart). Draw the privacy curtain between beds to minimize opportunities for close contact.

   - Change protective attire and perform hand hygiene between contact with patients in the same room, regardless of whether one or both patients are on droplet precautions

2. A mask is required when entering the room

3. Limit the movement/transport of patients from the room to essential purposes only. During transport, minimize the spread of droplets by placing a surgical mask on the patient, if possible, and asking the patient to follow respiratory hygiene/cough etiquette. No mask is required of persons transporting patients on droplet precautions.

FIGURE 8.3 • ISOLATION TECHNIQUES AND REQUIREMENTS (CONT.)

Contact Precautions

In addition to standard precautions, use contact precautions for specified patients known or suspected to be infected or colonized with epidemiologically important microorganisms that can be transmitted by direct contact with the patient (hand or skin-to-skin contact that occurs when performing patient care activities that require touching the patient's dry skin) or direct contact (touching) with environmental surfaces or patient care items in the environment.

1. A private room is preferable. When a private room is not available, cohort with a patient who has active infection or colonization with the same microorganism but no other infection. If it becomes necessary to place a patient on contact precautions in a room with a patient who is not infected or colonized with the same infectious agent:

   • Avoid placing with a patient who may have a condition that increases the risk of adverse outcome from infection or that may facilitate transmission (e.g., those who are imunocompromised, have open wounds, or have an anticipated length of stay).

   • Ensure that patients are physically separated (at least 3 ft. apart). Draw the privacy curtain between beds to minimize opportunities for direct contact.

   • Change protective attire and perform hand hygiene between contact with patients in the same room, regardless of whether one or both patients are on contact precautions.

2. Wear gloves when entering all contact precaution rooms. Change gloves during the course of caring for one patient and after contact with infective material. Remove gloves before leaving the patient's room.

3. Wash your hands immediately with alcohol hand rub or antimicrobial agent before leaving the patient's room. After glove removal and hand washing, ensure that hands do not touch potentially contaminated environmental surfaces or items in the patient's room to avoid transfer of microorganisms to other patients or environments. **Note:** Wash hands with soap and water if the patient has suspect or confirmed *Clostridium difficile*.

4. Wear a gown when entering all contact precaution rooms. After gown removal, ensure that clothing and skin do not contact potentially contaminated environmental surfaces that could result in possible transfer of microorganisms to other patients and surfaces.

FIGURE 8.3 • ISOLATION TECHNIQUES AND REQUIREMENTS (CONT.)

5. Wear a mask only to enter the room of patients suspected or known to have RSV or methicillin-resistant *Staphylococcus aureus* pneumonia

6. Limit the movement/transport of patients from the room for essential purposes only. During transport, ensure that infected or colonized areas of the patient's body are covered and contained. Remove and dispose of contaminated PPE in the patient's room and perform hand hygiene prior to leaving the room. Prior to transporting the patient on contact, don clean PPE. The patient's therapeutic needs may require therapy or activity outside of the room; in this case, the infection control committee may be consulted if questions or concerns arise.

7. When possible, dedicate the use of noncritical patient care equipment for each patient. If use of common equipment is necessary, then adequate cleaning and disinfection is required prior to the use for another patient.

8. Ensure that contact precaution rooms are prioritized for frequent cleaning (i.e., at least daily) with a focus on frequently touched surfaces (e.g., bedrails, over bed tables, bedside commodes, lavatory surfaces, doorknobs) and equipment in the immediate vicinity of the patient

   Note: All patients on precautions who must be transported out of their rooms will be handled on a case-by-case basis. For example, a patient who wants to be out of his or her room but does not have good patient hygiene or whose secretions cannot be contained should not be allowed to leave his or her room.

Reference
1. CDC Guideline for Isolation Precautions, 2007.

Source: Reprinted with permission form Libby Chinnes, RN, BSN, CIC, IC Solutions, LLC.

Cleaning, Disinfection, and Sterilization

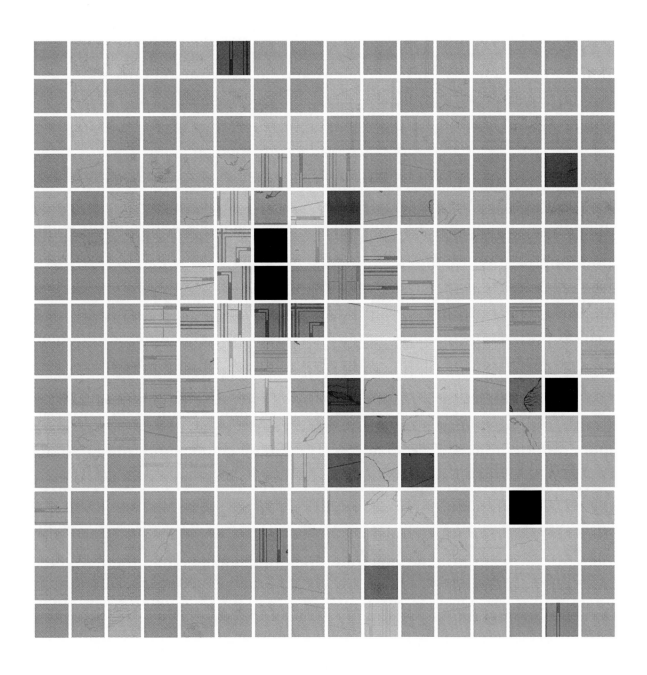

Cleaning, Disinfection, and Sterilization

Cleaning, disinfection, and sterilization processes essentially involve patient care equipment and the healthcare environment. For disinfection and sterilization to work, an item must be cleaned first. "Disinfection and sterilization are essential for ensuring that medical and surgical instruments do not transmit infectious pathogens to patients. Because sterilization of all patient care items is not necessary, healthcare policies must identify, primarily on the basis of the items' intended use, whether cleaning, disinfection, or sterilization is indicated," according to the Healthcare Infection Control Practices Advisory Committee (HICPAC) "Guideline for Disinfection and Sterilization in Healthcare Facilities, 2008."[1] Lack of compliance with proper processes has resulted in numerous outbreaks in healthcare settings. The infection preventionist (IP) plays a major role in product selection, educating staff members, and monitoring compliance with proper cleaning, disinfection, and sterilization processes. If you are a new IP, you will benefit greatly from spending time in your facility's central processing department to observe and learn firsthand about many of the topics covered in this chapter.

COMMON TERMINOLOGY

The following is a list of common terms you will encounter with cleaning, disinfection, and sterilization processes:

Cleaning: The removal of visible dust, soils, and any foreign material usually by manual means or mechanically by use of water with detergents or enzymatic products. An item must first be clean before it can be disinfected or sterilized.

Decontamination: A process that removes pathogens in order to render an item safe to handle, use, or discard

Disinfection: A process that eliminates many, or all, pathogens, except bacterial spores, on inanimate objects. In healthcare settings, this process is accomplished by chemicals or wet pasteurization

Pathogen: A disease-producing organism

Sterilization: A process that destroys or eliminates all forms of microbial life by physical or chemical means. In healthcare, the main sterilizing agents are steam under pressure, dry heat, ethylene oxide gas EtO, hydrogen peroxide gas plasma, and liquid chemicals.

Germicide: An agent that kills microorganisms, especially pathogens. This term encompasses antiseptics and disinfectants.

Antiseptic: Germicide applied to living tissues and skin. Examples include alcohol, povidone iodine, and chlorhexidine gluconate.

Vegetative bacteria: Bacteria without spores that usually can be readily inactivated by many types of germicides

Spore: A cell consisting of condensed cytoplasm and a nucleus surrounded by an impervious cell wall. Spores are relatively resistant to disinfectants, sterilants, and drying conditions.

Chemical sterilant: A disinfectant that kills spores with prolonged contact (three to 12 hours). At similar concentrations but shorter exposure times (e.g., 2% glutaraldehyde for 20 minutes), these high-level disinfectants will kill all organisms with the exception of large numbers of bacterial spores.

SPAULDING CLASSIFICATION SYSTEM

Decades ago, Earl Spaulding developed a rational process for determining how patient care items should be disinfected and sterilized. Classifications were denoted as critical, semicritical, and noncritical. This process is still used today.

Critical items

Critical items present a high risk of infection if contaminated and used on a patient because they enter sterile tissue or the vascular system and therefore need **sterilization**. Surgical instruments, cardiac catheters, and implants are some examples of critical items. Many items in this category may be purchased sterile or steam sterilized, if possible. If an item is heat-sensitive, EtO, hydrogen peroxide gas plasma, or liquid chemical sterilants are alternatives if other methods are not suitable. Germicides categorized as chemical sterilants include $\geq$ 2.4% glutaraldehyde-based formulations, 0.95% glutaraldehyde with 1.64% phenol/phenate, 7.5% stabilized hydrogen peroxide, 7.35% hydrogen peroxide with 0.23% peracetic acid, 0.2% peracetic acid, and 0.08% peracetic acid with 1% hydrogen peroxide. To successfully use a liquid chemical sterilant, you must clean the item first and follow all manufacturer instructions on use of the chemical. See the HICPAC/Centers for Disease Control and Prevention guidance, Table 1, Methods of Sterilization and Disinfection, for specific examples.

Semicritical items

Semicritical items contact mucous membranes or nonintact skin, and, therefore, a small number of spores is permissible. Semicritical items require, at a minimum, **high-level disinfection** using chemical disinfectants. High-level disinfection is the complete elimination of all microorganisms in or on an instrument, except for small numbers of bacterial spores. Glutaraldehyde, hydrogen peroxide, ortho-phthalaldehyde, and peracetic acid with hydrogen peroxide are approved by the FDA as high-level disinfectants. Some examples of semicritical items are:

- Respiratory therapy and anesthesia equipment
- Some endoscopes
- Laryngoscope blades
- Esophageal manometry probes
- Cystoscopes

Ideally, laparoscopes and arthroscopes entering sterile tissue should be sterilized between patients. However, there are no published reports of outbreaks resulting from these scopes when they are properly cleaned and undergo high-level disinfection. Rinsing endoscopes and channels with sterile water, filtered water, or tap water will prevent adverse effects associated with disinfectant retained in the endoscope (such as ac chemical-induced colitis). Items can be rinsed and flushed using sterile water after high-level disinfection to prevent contamination with organisms in tap water, such as nontuberculous mycobacteria, *Legionella,* or gram-negative bacilli such as *Pseudomonas.*

Intermediate-level disinfection inactivates *Mycobacterium tuberculosis,* vegetative bacteria, most viruses, and most fungi, but does not necessarily kill bacterial spores. Intermediate disinfectants include: 70%–90% ethyl or isopropyl alcohol, sodium hypochlorite, iodophors, and phenolics. Some items that may come in contact with nonintact skin for a brief time (e.g., hydrotherapy tanks) are usually considered noncritical surfaces and are disinfected with intermediate-level disinfectants.

Noncritical items

Noncritical items are those that come into contact with the protective intact skin but not mucous membranes. Noncritical items may be divided into two classes, such as noncritical patient care items (e.g., bedpans, blood pressure cuffs, computers, crutches) and noncritical environmental surfaces (e.g., bed rails, some food utensils, bedside tables, patient furniture, floors). **Low-level disinfectants** are appropriate for noncritical items and surfaces because these items pose no infection risk when used as noncritical items. Low-level disinfectants kill most vegetative bacteria, most fungi, and both lipid and nonlipid viruses; however, these disinfectants can not be relied on to kill resistant organisms such as Mycobacterium or spores. These disinfectants include 70%–90% ethyl or isopropyl alcohol, sodium hypochlorite, iodophors, phenolics, and quaternary ammonium compounds.

If you think of organisms on a ladder of resistance, as in Figure 9.1, with decreasing order of resistance to sterilization and disinfection, the top rung in the ladder would be bacterial spores, as these would be the most difficult organisms to kill (other than prions, such as those that cause Creutzfeldt-Jakob Disease). High-level disinfection would be a rung below sterilization, as it would kill all organisms, including Mycobacterium tuberculosis, except for bacterial spores. Intermediate- and low-level disinfection would follow on the lower rungs respectively.

IPs can use the Spaulding classification system to help decipher which process to use based on an item's intended use. It is critical to follow the manufacturer's guidelines for effectiveness and safety. You should also use personal protective equipment as appropriate.

Regulation

In the United States, healthcare chemical disinfectants are approved and regulated by two federal agencies: the Environmental Protection Agency (EPA) and the FDA.

The EPA regulates:

- Pesticides (including disinfectants and sterilants used on inanimate objects and environmental surfaces)
- Medical waste incinerators

The FDA regulates:

- Medical devices, including reuse
- Drugs for human/animal use
- High-level disinfectants and sterilants
- Blood products

In general, the EPA regulates disinfectants and sterilants used on environmental surfaces, but not those used on critical or semicritical medical devices; the FDA regulates the latter. The IP should make sure that the facility is using EPA-approved disinfectants by noting the EPA product number on the product label. The IP should also be included, per The Joint Commission, in determining any product selection criteria that affects decontamination, cleaning, disinfection, and sterilization practices.

Note: Although disinfectants and sterilants are regulated, the IP should also be aware that recommendations are available through the CDC to the public and healthcare personnel regarding current science and which chemicals might be most effective in particular situations.

DISINFECTION

An ideal disinfectant:

- Kills a wide array of organisms (has a broad spectrum)
- Acts quickly
- Is a good cleaner
- Is compatible with all surfaces
- Is nontoxic
- Is not affected by environmental factors, such as water hardness
- Has a residual effect
- Is soluble in water
- Is stable in concentration and use-dilution
- Is odorless
- Is user-friendly
- Is economical[2]

That said, thus far, there is no ideal disinfectant. They all have advantages and disadvantages. Refer to the CDC's "Guideline for Disinfection and Sterilization in Healthcare Facilities, 2008" for a closer look at each chemical.

Remember, follow the label and manufacturer's instructions for dilution and use. Cross contamination can occur if disinfectants or antiseptics are topped off (i.e., more product added to residual in container to fill the container to the top).

High-level disinfection of instruments

Instruments or endoscopes are usually soaked after use in enzymatic detergents to prevent blood and soils, which harbor microorganisms, from drying on the instruments. A healthcare worker wearing the proper attire should clean the instruments before either manual or automated disinfection. Disassemble each instrument as completely as possible and immerse it in the enzymatic solution during cleaning in order to reach all crevices and surfaces. Rinse and dry items. Discard the enzymatic solution after each use, as it will not inhibit microbial growth.

Immerse the "cleaned" instrument in a covered container of prepared high-level disinfectant. Make sure you thoroughly rinse and dry the instruments before placing them in the high-level disinfectant to avoid diluting the disinfectant. Federal regulations require you to follow the FDA-cleared label claim for each specific high-level disinfectant. The FDA-cleared labels for high-level disinfection with > 2% glutaraldehyde at 25°C range from 20 to 90 minutes, depending on the product used. Several scientific studies and professional organizations support the efficacy of > 2% glutaraldehyde for 20 minutes at 20°C. Facilities that choose to apply the 20-minute duration at 20°C base their decision on the type IA (strongly recommended) recommendation in the July 2003 Society for Healthcare Epidemiology of America position paper, "Multi-Society Guideline for Reprocessing Flexible Gastrointestinal Endoscopes."[3] The 20-minute claim assumes that the item has been adequately precleaned, whereas the FDA-cleared label claim adds an extra layer of safety for an item that may not have been adequately cleaned.[4]

Rinse disinfected instruments with sterile, filtered, or tap water as appropriate, and then dry them. If the instrument is an endoscope, make sure you thoroughly immerse all channels in the disinfectant, rinse them with water, and then rinse the endoscope with 70%–90% ethyl or isopropyl alcohol and purge with forced air to remove risk of contamination with waterborne organisms.

You should routinely test liquid sterilants/ high-level disinfectants to ensure that there is a minimal effective concentration of the active ingredient. Test solutions each day of use (or more frequently) using the appropriate chemical indicator (e.g., glutaraldehyde chemical indicator to test minimal effective concentration of glutaraldehyde) and document the results. Dispose of the solution if the chemical indicator shows the concentration is less than the minimum effective concentration, even if you have not exceeded the reuse life recommended by the manufacturer. Do not reuse liquid sterilants/high-level disinfectants beyond the reuse life recommended by the manufacturer (e.g., 14 days for ortho-phthalaldehyde). Make sure workers use these chemicals in properly ventilated areas to prevent exposures to potentially toxic fumes (e.g., glutaraldehye).

Provide healthcare personnel who reprocess endoscopes with device-specific reprocessing instructions to ensure proper cleaning and high-level disinfection or sterilization. Perform worker competency testing on a regular basis.

Tip: William A. Rutala, MD, maintains a helpful Web site on disinfection and sterilization, *www. disinfectionandsterilization.org.* The site hosts a wide variety of resources, including PowerPoint lectures, the most recent updates on disinfection and sterilization processes, an endoscope reprocessing competency checklist, free reprocessing posters from manufacturers, the FDA-cleared sterilant and high-level disinfectant list, as well as a current list of EPA-registered antimicrobials.

STERILIZATION AND MONITORING

Steam is the preferred method of sterilization for critical instruments that cannot be damaged by heat or moisture. You must follow the sterilization times, temperatures, and other operating parameters (e.g., gas concentration and humidity) recommended by the manufacturers of the instruments, the sterilizer, and the container or wrap used, as well as those from guidelines published by government agencies and professional organizations (e.g., the Association for the Advancement of Medical Instrumentation [AAMI] and the Association of periOperative Registered Nurses [AORN]).

If critical patient care equipment is heat- or moisture-sensitive, low-temperature sterilization technologies, such as EtO or hydrogen peroxide gas plasma, are recommended for sterilization. EtO-sterilized items require aeration before use on a patient. Sterilization using the peracetic acid immersion system can be used to sterilize heat-sensitive immersible items, but critical items sterilized in this fashion must be used immediately (i.e., just-in-time sterilization), as they are not protected from contamination. This also means that long-term storage of these items is not possible. Dry heat sterilization (e.g., 340°F for 60 minutes) is another method of sterilization that you can use to sterilize items such as powders and oils, which can sustain high temperatures. In all cases, you must use packaging compatible with the chosen sterilization process. A comparison of the different sterilization technologies is listed in Figure 9.1.

FIGURE 9.1 • MICROORGANISMS: ORDER OF RESISTANCE

This figure shows the decreasing order of resistance of microorganisms to disinfection and sterilization and the level of disinfection or sterilization.

RESISTANT

Microorganisms	Level of Sterilization
Prions (Creutzfeldt-Jakob Disease)	Prion reprocessing
Bacterial spores (*Bacillus atrophaeus*)	Sterilization
Coccidia (*Cryptosporidium*)	Sterilization
Mycobacteria (*M. tuberculosis, M. terrae*)	High
Nonlipid or small viruses (polio, coxsackie)	Intermediate
Fungi (*Aspergillus, Candida*)	Intermediate
Vegetative bacteria (*S. aureus, P. aeruginosa*)	Low
Lipid or medium-sized viruses (HIV, herpes, hepatitis B)	Low

SUSCEPTIBLE

Source: William A. Rutala, Ph.D., M.P.H., David J. Weber, M.D., M.P.H., and the Healthcare Infection Control Practices Advisory Committee (HICPAC), "Guideline for Disinfection and Sterilization in Healthcare Facilities, 2008," Centers for Disease Control and Prevention, *www.cdc.gov/ncidod/dhqp/pdf/guidelines/Disinfection_Nov_2008.pdf* (accessed September 3, 2009).

Types of indicators

Whatever sterilization method you use, you must monitor the process. According to the CDC, you should monitor each sterilized load with **mechanical indicators** (i.e., time, pressure, and temperature) as well as **chemical indicators** (internal and external). If any of these "first alarm" indicators suggest an inadequate process, do not use the processed item, as it may not be sterile. Mechanical indicators are displayed with each load on the sterilizer gauge, printout, or graph. Chemical indicators, placed on the outside of each package, signal that the item has been exposed to sterilization—this does not mean that the item is sterile. These indicators should also be placed on the inside of each package to verify that steam penetration occurred.

There are two basic types of steam sterilizers (i.e., autoclaves): gravity-displacement and high-speed prevacuum sterilizers. Gravity-displacement sterilizers admit steam at the top or sides of the chamber, and gravity forces the air out through a drain vent at the bottom of the sterilizer. Penetration time into porous items is prolonged, as there is incomplete air removal. The vacuum sterilizer is similar but uses a vacuum pump to pull air out of the chamber before it admits steam. Unremoved air will interfere with steam contact and sterilization of the load. Perform a daily Bowie-Dick test only in an empty prevacuum sterilizer to check for complete air removal. If the sterilizer does not pass the Bowie-Dick test, do not use it until it is inspected by the sterilizer maintenance personnel and passes another Bowie-Dick test.

Biological indicators are the closest monitor of the sterilization process, as they measure the process directly by using the most resistant microorganisms (i.e., *Bacillus* spores), and not by merely testing the physical and chemical conditions. If the *Bacillus* spores are killed, this strongly implies that other potential pathogens in the load have been killed. The CDC recommends using biological indicators at least weekly, but preferably daily, with an FDA-cleared commercial preparation of spores (e.g., *Geobacillus stearothermophilus* for steam) intended specifically for the type and cycle parameters of the sterilizer. The CDC also recommends using biological indicators with every load containing implantable items and that the items are quarantined, whenever possible, until the biologic indicator is negative.

Figure 9.2 outlines how to handle a positive biological indicator.

FIGURE 9.2 • BIOLOGICAL INDICATORS

Handling of a positive biological indicator with steam sterilization

- After a single positive biological indicator (BI) with a steam sterilizer, recall only implantable objects unless the sterilizer was set to an inappropriate cycle or maintenance personnel determine that the sterilizer or procedure are defective

- If additional BIs remain positive, consider items nonsterile; recall any items dating back to the implicated load(s) and reprocess

Handling of a positive biological indicator with sterilization other than steam

- After a single positive BI with sterilization methods other than steam sterilization, consider all items nonsterile, dating back to the last negative BI noted

- If possible, retrieve nonsterile items and reprocess

Source: William A. Rutala, Ph.D., M.P.H., David J. Weber, M.D., M.P.H., and the Healthcare Infection Control Practices Advisory Committee (HICPAC), "Guideline for Disinfection and Sterilization in Healthcare Facilities, 2008," Centers for Disease Control and Prevention, *www.cdc.gov/ncidod/dhqp/pdf/guidelines/Disinfection_Nov_2008.pdf* (accessed September 3, 2009).

Flash sterilization

Flash sterilization is a modification of the steam sterilization process in which the flashed item is placed in an open tray (unwrapped) or in a specially designed, covered, rigid container to allow for rapid penetration of steam. It is an acceptable form of sterilization, but *only* for urgently needed items that will be used immediately (e.g., a dropped instrument). It is not a substitute for an inadequate inventory of instruments or to be used for the sake of convenience. When flashing an item, ensure that you clean it properly first. Also use the item close to the point of sterilization. Monitor all flashed cycles with mechanical, chemical, and biological indicators, and be sure to protect flashed items from contamination during transport. Never flash implantable items unless it is unavoidable due to the potential for serious infections. AORN, AAMI and the Joint Commission all have guidelines on flashing implants. Your facility should keep manufacturer's instructions for flashing near sterilizers and maintain logs of all items it flashes for formal review as part of its performance improvement practice.

Reuse of single-use medical devices

The FDA released a guidance document in 2000 about single-use devices reprocessed by third parties or hospitals.[5] Because the reuse of single-use devices involves regulatory, ethical, medical, legal, and economic concerns and has been extremely controversial for more than two decades, the FDA states that hospitals or third-party reprocessors that choose to reprocess single-use items will be considered "manufacturers" and regulated in the same manner. A reused single-use device will have to comply with the same regulatory requirements of the device when it was originally manufactured. A hospital's choices are: not to reprocess, outsource to a third-party reprocessor, or reprocess per the FDA document. The CDC's "Guideline for Disinfection and Sterilization in Healthcare Facilities, 2008," states that the "FDA guidance document does not apply to permanently implantable pacemakers, hemodialyzers, opened but unused single-use devices, or healthcare settings other than acute care hospitals. The reuse of single-use medical devices continues to be an evolving area of regulations. For this reason, healthcare workers should refer to the FDA for the latest guidance *(www.fda.gov."*

Storage

After sterilization, handle instruments aseptically to prevent contamination. Sterile supplies should be stored eight to 10 inches from the floor, 18 inches from a sprinkler head, and two inches from outside walls. Make sure you use a solid bottom shelf; the ideal spot is a closed or covered cabinet, but open shelves are acceptable. *Note:* Do not store anything under the sink where items may get wet and contaminated. Do not use any item that you suspect is contaminated, and be sure to return that item to your central processing department for reprocessing. If your facility uses time-related storage of sterile items, label the pack with an expiration date at the time of sterilization. Once this date expires, reprocess the pack. Many facilities have adopted an "event-related" sterilization policy, which states that an item is sterile indefinitely unless an event happens to compromise the packaging (e.g., a tear, moisture, or a puncture).

TIPS ON CLEANING AND DISINFECTING

Physical cleaning is important to remove soil and reduce the microbial load in a healthcare facility. Remember, it is critical to follow the manufacturer's instructions for the items your facility uses. Pay particular attention to the most soiled and/or contaminated areas such as the floor and hospital surfaces, especially in patient rooms. Clean housekeeping surfaces (e.g., floors and tabletops) on a regular basis, when spills occur, and when these surfaces are visibly soiled. Disinfect or otherwise clean other environmental surfaces on a regular basis and when visibly soiled. Wet mopping is the preferred cleaning method for floors, as dry sweeping disseminates organisms (and should be avoided). Prepare disinfecting or detergent solutions as needed and replace these with fresh solution frequently (e.g., replace floor mopping solution every three patient rooms and change no less often than at 60-minute intervals),[6] according to the facility's policy, per the CDC guidelines. You may also use a one-step process with an EPA-registered hospital disinfectant/detergent.

The following are additional strategies:[7]

- Launder and dry mop heads and cleaning cloths at least daily to prevent contamination

- Spot-clean walls when spills/splashes occur

- Never use high-level disinfectants on noncritical surfaces

- Wet dust horizontal surfaces regularly (e.g., daily or three times per week, etc.) using clean cloths moistened with an EPA-registered hospital disinfectant or detergent

Blood spills

For spills of blood or other potentially infectious material (OPIM), the Occupational Safety and Health Administration requires the use of personal protective equipment and one of the following:

- An EPA-registered tuberculocidal agent

- A registered germicide with specific label claims for HIV or hepatitis B virus

- A freshly diluted hypochlorite solution[8]

If your facility uses sodium hypochlorite solutions, the CDC guidelines recommend a 1:100 dilution (e.g., 1:100 dilution of a 5.25%–6.15% sodium hypochlorite provides 525–615 ppm of available chlorine) to decontaminate nonporous surfaces after a small spill (e.g., < 10 mL). If a spill involves large amounts (e.g., > 10 mL) of blood or OPIM, or involves a culture spill in the laboratory, use a 1:10 dilution for the first application of hypochlorite solution before cleaning to reduce the infection risk during cleaning in the event of a sharps injury. Follow this decontamination process with a terminal disinfection, using a 1:100 dilution of sodium hypochlorite.

If the spill contains large amounts of blood or body fluids, clean the visible matter with disposable, absorbent material and discard the contaminated materials in an appropriate, labeled biohazard container.

Clostridium difficile

When a facility is experiencing high endemic rates of *Clostridium difficile*, or an outbreak has occurred, use dilute solutions of 5.25%–6.15% sodium hypochlorite (e.g., 1:10 dilution of household bleach) for routine environmental disinfection per CDC guidelines.

Bloodborne and emerging pathogens

Compliance with the disinfection and sterilization practices noted in the CDC guidelines in this chapter is adequate to sterilize or disinfect instruments or devices contaminated with blood or other body fluids from persons infected with bloodborne pathogens or emerging pathogens, with the exception of prions. See the specific guidelines for details on prions.[9]

For more information

Table 6 in the "Guideline for Disinfection and Sterilization in Healthcare Facilities, 2008" summarizes the advantages and disadvantages of commonly used sterilization technologies. It is available at *www.cdc.gov/ncidod/dhqp/pdf/guidelines/Disinfection_Nov_2008.pdf.*

More on sterilization and disinfection can be found in the following resources:

- FDA, *www.fda.gov*
- EPA, *www.epa.gov/oppad001*
- CDC, *www.cdc.gov/ncidod/dhqp/sterile.html*
- University of North Carolina in Chapel Hill, *www.disinfectionandsterilization.org*

REFERENCES

1. William A. Rutala, David J. Weber, "Guideline for Disinfection and Sterilization in Healthcare Facilities, 2008," Centers for Disease Control and Prevention, *www.cdc.gov/ncidod/dhqp/pdf/guidelines/Disinfection_Nov_2008.pdf* (accessed September 3, 2009).

2. Ibid.

3. D.B. Nelson, W.R. Jarvis, W.A. Rutula, et al., "Multi-Society Guideline for Reprocessing Flexible Gastro-intestinal Endoscopes," *Infection Control and Hospital Epidemiology* 24 (2003): 532–537.

4. William A. Rutala, David J. Weber, "Guideline for Disinfection and Sterilization in Healthcare Facilities, 2008," Centers for Disease Control and Prevention, *www.cdc.gov/ncidod/dhqp/pdf/guidelines/Disinfection_Nov_2008.pdf* (accessed September 3, 2009).

5. "Enforcement Priorities for Single-Use Devices Reprocessed by Third Parties and Hospitals," Food and Drug Administration, *www.fda.gov/MedicalDevices/DeviceRegulationandGuidance/GuidanceDocuments/ucm107164.htm* (accessed September 3, 2009).

6. William A. Rutala, David J. Weber, "Guideline for Disinfection and Sterilization in Healthcare Facilities, 2008," Centers for Disease Control and Prevention, *www.cdc.gov/ncidod/dhqp/pdf/guidelines/Disinfection_Nov_2008.pdf* (accessed September 3, 2009).

7. Sehulster, Lynne, Chinn, Raymond, "Guidelines for Environmental Infection Control in Health-Care Facilities," Recommendations of CDC and the Healthcare Infection Control Practices Advisory Committee (HICPAC), June 6, 2003/52 (RR-10); 1–42.

8. OSHA 29 *CFR* 1910.1030 § d.4.ii. A memorandum 2/28/97; compliance document [CPL] 2-2.44D [11/99].

9. William A. Rutala, David J. Weber, "Guideline for Disinfection and Sterilization in Healthcare Facilities, 2008," Centers for Disease Control and Prevention, *www.cdc.gov/ncidod/dhqp/pdf/guidelines/Disinfection_Nov_2008.pdf* (accessed September 3, 2009).

Employee Health and Employee Education

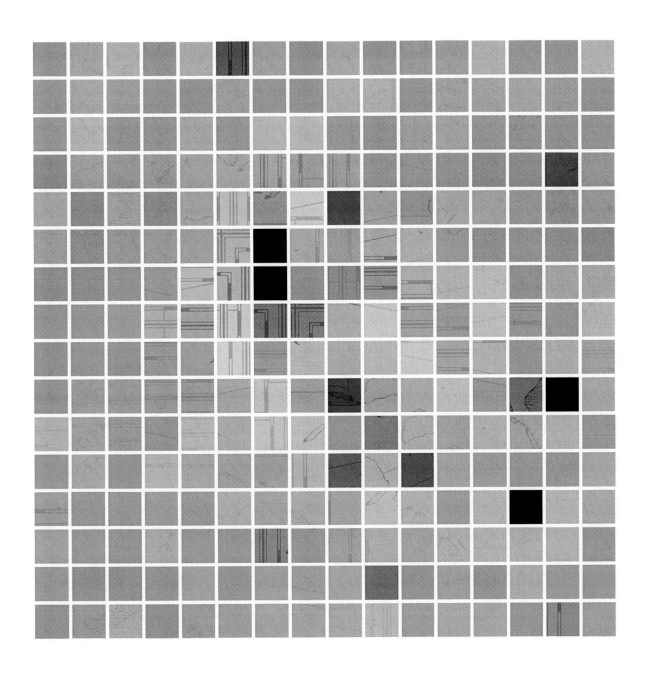

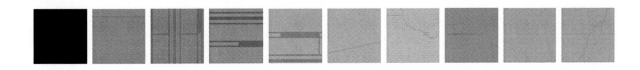

Employee Health and Employee Education

The health of a facility's employees plays a major role in infection prevention and control. One of the goals of an infection prevention and control program in any setting is to protect not just the health of patients but also that of employees.[1] The infection preventionist (IP) may hold a dual role, leading both the IP and employee health departments in many facilities. If you are a full-time IP, you will need to communicate and collaborate with the employee health professional on a regular basis.

The Centers for Disease Control and Prevention (CDC) produced a helpful resource for IPs as well as employee health professionals entitled "Guideline for Infection Control in Health Care Personnel, 1998" (*www.cdc.gov*). IPs will need to stay abreast of current issues in employee health through the CDC's *Morbidity and Mortality Weekly Report* (*MMWR*). For example, newer information on the varicella vaccine and tuberculosis has been published since the 1998 employee health guidelines. By searching the Internet for your topic or skimming the *MMWR* back issues, one can see updates in information to be added to the basic set of 1998 guidelines.

A basic tenet of any infection control or employee health program is education of your employees. Employees are more likely to comply with measures if they understand why they are being asked to do so. In addition, The Joint Commission is now also very prescriptive on what employees must be taught in terms of infection prevention and control.

EMPLOYEE HEALTH

First of all, who are your employees? Per the CDC guidelines, healthcare personnel are "all paid and unpaid persons working in healthcare settings (in and outside of hospitals) who have the potential for exposures to infectious materials, including body substances, contaminated medical supplies and equipment, contaminated environmental surfaces, or contaminated air."[2] Don't forget about volunteers, students, contract workers, and licensed independent practitioners, as these folks may also be the weak link in the chain of transmitting infection if not vaccinated properly or handled appropriately after an exposure. For example, a pediatric resident who may have been overlooked in an exposure incident may not be immune to varicella and may actually spread the disease in the early symptomatic stage as he or she rounds through your facility. Or a volunteer who comes to work with influenza-like symptoms may be the index case for the start of influenza in your organization. Your facility may not have to address all these directly, as in the case of students, but should have documentation that these healthcare workers have the proper immunizations, for example, as part of their contract before working in your facility.

ELEMENTS OF AN EMPLOYEE HEALTH SERVICE

The following are components of an effective employee health program:

- **Coordination with other departments.** Employee health services involves all employees, and, therefore, coordination must occur with all departments. Collaboration with the IP is crucial on surveillance and trending of specific infections in staff members, exposures to infectious diseases in and out of the workplace, and restrictions of the ill or contagious employee.

- **Medical evaluations.** Before job placement, a health inventory is usually conducted. Included in the evaluation is an assessment of immunization status of the worker as well as predisposing conditions for infections. Some facilities may even conduct employee physical exams and lab tests based on the inventory. The facility may find it helpful and cost-effective to screen for some vaccine-preventable diseases. These evaluations are redone periodically, such as annually or when an employee receives a new job assignment.

- **Health and safety education.** All employees need infection control education and training. The IP and the employee health professional can collaborate to conduct this training separately or jointly. Specific diseases or conditions in employees may require individualized training in order for employees to perform their duties safely.

- **Immunization programs.** Immunization programs are the most cost-effective means to protect employees and patients from infectious diseases. The U.S. Public Health Service's Advisory Committee on Immunization Practices provides national guidelines on vaccines and postexposure prophylaxis for healthcare workers. (See the "Vaccines strongly recommended for healthcare workers" sidebar).

Vaccines strongly[†] recommended for healthcare workers[3,4]

Hepatitis B vaccine*

Annual influenza vaccine

Measles vaccine

Mumps vaccine

Rubella vaccine

Varicella vaccine

Tdap vaccine (tetanus, diphtheria, and pertussis)

† Other agents are available for special circumstances
* Also required per the Occupational Safety and Health Administration for healthcare workers at risk of exposure to blood and body fluids

---

- Management of job-related illnesses and exposures to infectious diseases, including policies for work. Employee health exists primarily to diagnose and manage job-related illnesses and handle employee exposures. (See the "Diseases for which postexposure prophylaxis may be indicated for healthcare personnel" sidebar.) This may involve only one employee or numerous staff members, as in an outbreak. The IP may do the follow-up, or he or she may only follow up on patient exposures, and the employee health professional may follow up on employees. Employee follow-up may need the assistance of department directors to look at staffing assignments and patient charts to determine which employees were potentially exposed and to have them report to employee health.

Diseases for which postexposure prophylaxis may be indicated for healthcare personnel[‡5,6]

Diphtheria

Hepatitis A

Hepatitis B

HIV

Meningococcal disease

Pertussis

Rabies

Varicella zoster virus

‡ Check the most current *MMWR* and *American Academy of Pediatric Red Book* for specifics on postexposure prophylaxis

---

- Restrictions for infected or exposed personnel. Sometimes to prevent infections from spreading, employee health must restrict workers from their duties and the healthcare facility. Exclusion policies should state who may exclude personnel from duty and encourage personnel to report exposures and specific signs and symptoms without fear of penalization.[7] (See Figure 10.1.)

- Counseling services for personnel about infection risks related to employment or special conditions. Individualized counseling of employees is critical to allay their fears and provide them with current information on exposure management, the risks and benefits of postexposure prophylaxis, information on infectious diseases, and measures to protect themselves and their families from infections.

- Maintenance and confidentiality of personnel health records. Employees should have personnel employee health records with their health inventory, immunization status, any screening tests ordered, and documentation of the management of exposures and illnesses. This information should be maintained confidentially and in accordance with all regulations, such as Occupational Safety and Health Administration (OSHA) recordkeeping standards. However, personnel may review their individual records. A computerized personnel database should be maintained to allow tracking of immunization status, for example, as well as trends in employee illnesses.

FIGURE 10.1 • SUGGESTED WORK RESTRICTIONS FOR INFECTED PERSONNEL[1]

Disease/problem	Work restriction	Duration
Conjunctivitis	Restrict from patient contact and contact with the patient's environment	Until discharge ceases
Cytomegalovirus infections	No restriction	
Diarrheal diseases:		
• Acute stage (diarrhea with other symptoms)	Restrict from patient contact, contact with the environment, or food handling	Until symptoms resolve
• Convalescent stage	Restrict from care of high-risk patients	Until symptoms resolve; consult with local and state health authorities regarding need for negative stool stool cultures
Diphtheria	Exclude from duty	Until antimicrobial therapy completed and two cultures obtained > 24 hours apart are negative
Enteroviral infections	Restrict from care of infants, neonates, and immunocompromised patients and their environments	Until symptoms resolve
Hepatitis A	Restrict from patient contact, contact with patient's environment, and food handling	Until seven days after onset of jaundice
• Personnel with acute or chronic hepatitis B surface antigenemia who do not perform exposure-prone procedures	No restriction.* Refer to state regulations; standard Precautions should always be observed	
• Personnel with acute or chronic hepatitis B e. antigenemia who perform exposure-prone procedures	Do not perform exposure-prone invasive procedures until counsel from an expert review panel has been sought; panel should review and recommend procedures the worker can perform, taking into account specific procedure as well as skill and techniques of worker; refer to state regulations	Until hepatitis B e. antigenemia is negative

FIGURE 10.1 • SUGGESTED WORK RESTRICTIONS FOR INFECTED PERSONNEL (CONT.)

Disease/problem	Work restriction	Duration
Hepatitis C	No recommendation	
Herpes simplex		
• Genital	No restriction	
• Hands (Herpetic Whitlow)	Restrict from patient contact and contact with the patient's environment	Until lesions are gone
• Orofacial	Evaluate for need to restrict from care of high-risk patients	
HIV	Do not perform exposure-prone invasive procedures until counsel from an expert review panel has been sought; panel should review and recommend procedures the worker can perform, taking into account specific procedure as well as skill and technique of the worker; standard precautions should always be observed; refer to state regulations	
Measles		
• Active	Exclude from duty	Until seven days after the rash appears
• Postexposure (susceptible personnel)	Exclude from duty	From fifth day after first exposure through 21st day after last exposure and/or four days after rash appears
Meningococcal infections	Exclude from duty	Until 24 hours after start of effective therapy
Mumps		
• Active	Exclude from duty	Until nine days after onset of parotitis
• Postexposure (susceptible personnel)	Exclude from duty	From 12th day after first exposure through 26th day after last exposure or until nine days after onset of parotitis
Pediculosis	Restrict from patient contact	Until treated and observed to be free of adult and immature lice

FIGURE 10.1 • SUGGESTED WORK RESTRICTIONS FOR INFECTED PERSONNEL (CONT.)

Disease/problem	Work restriction	Duration
Pertussis		
• Active	Exclude from duty	From beginning of catarrhal stage through third week after onset of paroxysms or until five days after start of effective antimicrobial therapy
• Postexposure (asymptomatic personnel)	No restriction, prophylaxis recommended	
• Postexposure (symptomatic personnel)	Exclude from duty	Until five days after start of effective antimicrobial therapy
Rubella		
• Active	Exclude from duty	Until five days after rash appears
• Postexposure (susceptible personnel)	Exclude from duty	From seventh day after first exposure through 21st day after last exposure
Scabies	Restrict from patient contact	Until cleared by medical evaluation
***Staphylococcus aureus* infection**		
• Active, draining skin lesions	Restrict from contact with patients and patient's environment or food handling	Until lesions have resolved
• Carrier state	No restriction, unless personnel are epidemiologically linked to transmission of the organism	
Streptococcal infection, Group A	Restrict from patient care, contact with patient's environment, or food handling	Until 24 hours after adequate treatment started
Tuberculosis		
• Active disease	Exclude from duty	Until proved noninfectious
• Purified protein derivative converter	No restriction	

| FIGURE 10.1 • SUGGESTED WORK RESTRICTIONS FOR INFECTED PERSONNEL (CONT.) |||
Disease/problem	Work restriction	Duration
Varicella		
• Active	Exclude from duty	Until all lesions dry and crust
• Postexposure	Exclude from duty	From 10th day after 1st exposure through the 21st day (28th day if VZIG given) after last exposure
Zoster		
• Localized in healthy person	Cover lesions; restrict from care of high-risk patients†	Until all lesions dry and crust
• Generalized or localized in immuno-suppressed person	Restrict from patient contact	Until all lesions dry and crust
• Postexposure (suscep-tible personnel)	Restrict from patient contact	From 10th day after first exposure through 21st day (28th day if VZIG given) after last exposure or, if varicella occurs, until all lesions dry and crust
Viral respiratory infections, acute febrile	Consider excluding from the care of high-risk patients‡ or contact with their environment during community outbreak of respiratory syncytial virus and influenza	Until acute symptoms resolve
* Unless epidemiologically linked to transmission of infection		
† Those susceptible to varicella and who are at increased risk of complications of varicella, such as neonates and immunocompromised persons of any age		
‡ High-risk patients as defined by the ACIP for complications of influenza		

Source: CDC, *www.cdc.gov.*

OTHER EMPLOYEE HEALTH ISSUES

In general, pregnant healthcare personnel do not have an increased risk for acquiring infections in the workplace and should strictly follow standard precautions with all patients as well as isolation precautions when indicated. Females of childbearing age should also be strongly encouraged to receive vaccinations for vaccine-preventable diseases before pregnancy.

Due to the nature of their work and practices such as mouth pipetting, aerosolization of specimens, and percutaneous injury, laboratory personnel remain at risk for occupational exposure and acquisition of infectious agents. Lab workers who may be exposed to infectious agents need to be very informed about the risks and measures to prevent exposure such as biosafety procedures, immunization, and postexposure prophylaxis, when indicated.

The 1990 Ryan White Comprehensive AIDS Resources Emergency Act requires each state to establish notification systems to inform emergency-response employees (including emergency medical technicians and firefighters) when they have been exposed to an emergency medical patient with an infectious, potentially fatal disease such as HIV or meningococcemia. This is a good reminder to watch for any personnel transporting this type of patient, as their agency needs to be notified of potential exposures.

EMPLOYEE EDUCATION[8,9]

A critical part of employee health is employee education on infection prevention and control. The employee health professional and the infection preventionist can share training sessions and collaborate on information needed by the staff members and providers for their protection as well as that of their patients. The following are only a few of the topics which should be covered:

- Hand hygiene

- Manner in which infections are spread and importance of complying with Standard and Transmission-Based Precautions

- Tuberculosis control

- Importance of reporting certain illnesses or conditions (whether work-related or acquired outside of work) such as generalized rash or skin lesions that are vesicular, pustular, or weeping; jaundice; illnesses that do not resolve within a designated period (e.g., a cough that persists for >2 weeks, gastrointestinal illness, or febrile illness with fever of >103°F lasting >2 days); and hospitalizations resulting from febrile or other contagious diseases

- Reporting exposure to blood and body fluids

- Importance of personnel screening, immunization, and health and hygiene maintenance

- Site-specific protocols

- Therapy

- Opportunity for questions and answers

According to OSHA, training must also be conducted for employees on bloodborne pathogens and tuberculosis. A synopsis follows:

Bloodborne Pathogens Exposure Control Plan Training includes:

- A copy of the OSHA bloodborne pathogens standard and your exposure control plan

- Symptoms of bloodborne diseases as well as how hepatitis B, C, and HIV are transmitted

- Tasks that could involve blood or body fluid exposures

- Methods of prevention such as engineering controls (including needleless devices and safety needles), work practices such as use of Standard Precautions, and personal protective equipment (PPE)

- PPE types, uses, location, removal, disposal

- Hepatitis B vaccine: efficacy, safety, method of administration, the benefits of being vaccinated, offered free of charge on-site

- Body fluid spill actions

- Exposure incident (what to do and where to report) along with postexposure evaluation

- Signs and labels and/or color-coding

- Opportunity for questions and answers with knowledgeable trainer

Tuberculosis Exposure Control Plan Training includes:

- Symptoms of TB and its epidemiology in the your setting

- Mode of transmission

- Proper isolation including use of negative air pressure rooms and PPE

- Signage advising respiratory hygiene and cough etiquette

- Tuberculin skin test screening based on risk assessment and state licensing regulations

- Handling of TB exposures

All of these list items need to be covered in new employee orientation and annual updates. Since some of the information does not change, be sure to use different forms of training, such as lectures, small group discussions, poster sessions, games, videos, pamphlets, an infection prevention fair, a scenario-based situation involving a "room full of errors," self-paced computer instructional booklet, etc. See Figure 10.2 and 10.3 for samples of real-life examples of employee education. Let your imagination run wild, just don't forget to use a knowledgeable person so he or she can answer questions at the end of the session as required per OSHA. Also, the basics of infection prevention and control never go out of style in any educational effort, so remember to focus on:

- Hand hygiene

- Standard precautions and cough etiquette

- Safe injection practices

- Isolation precautions

- Cleaning, disinfection, and sterilization

FIGURE 10.2 • SAMPLE INFECTION CONTROL COMPETENCY TEST

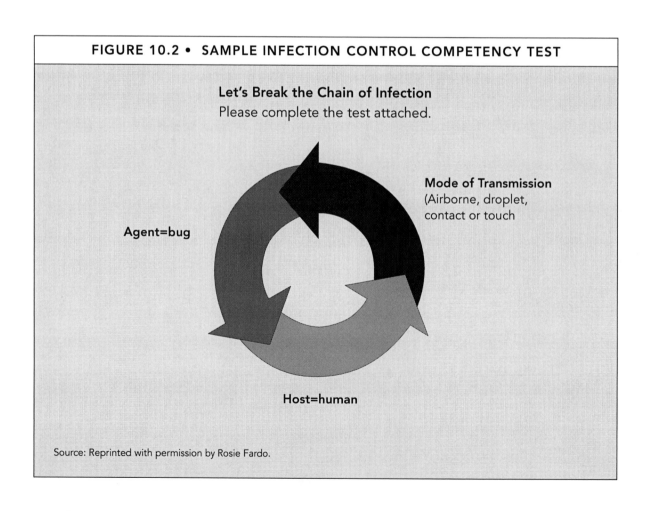

Let's Break the Chain of Infection
Please complete the test attached.

Mode of Transmission
(Airborne, droplet, contact or touch

Agent=bug

Host=human

Source: Reprinted with permission by Rosie Fardo.

FIGURE 10.2 • SAMPLE INFECTION CONTROL COMPETENCY TEST (CONT.)

Name: _____   Department: _____

Test Score: _____
Passing test score is 84.

Circle the answer that applies.

1. Hand antisepsis using alcohol-based hand rubs should be used in the following clinical situations:

    a. After contact with patient's blood

    b. After exposure to *C. difficile*

    c. Before and after caring for the patient

    d. All the above

2. The following is true of alcohol-based hand rubs:

    a. They require more time to use than soap and water

    b. They are not effective

    c. They are more effective against 99% of bacterial and viral organisms

    d. They dry your hands out

3. In order to protect employees from bloodborne pathogens, the hospital must provide employees with engineering controls, work practice controls, and PPE. Which of the following is **NOT** an example of PPE?

    a. Mask

    b. Gowns

    c. Scrubs

    d. Gloves

    e. Face shield

4. PPE is worn any time it is anticipated that you will be coming in contact with blood/body fluids or nonintact skin.

    a. True

    b. False

FIGURE 10.2 • SAMPLE INFECTION CONTROL COMPETENCY TEST (CONT.)

5. Gloves do not need to be changed between different body sites on the same patient.

    a. True

    b. False

6. Nursing has the authority and responsibility to implement precautions according to the hospital policy.

    a. True

    b. False

7. A patient comes to the facility complaining of night sweats, cough, bloody sputum and weight loss—the classic symptoms of TB. The patient is to be isolated in a negative pressure room *but no room is immediately available*. What is the *first* thing to do?

    a. Ask the patient to wear a surgical mask

    b. Nothing—the patient should not have to be moved twice

    c. Place the patient in a private room

    d. Call the employee health department and have the patient fitted with a TB respirator

8. You work in a department with a negative pressure room and are therefore required to be fit-tested to wear a TB respirator. Which of the following statements about respirators is *false*?

    a. You must be annually fit-tested and approved by the employee health department to wear an N95 respirator when caring for a TB patient

    b. You must perform a fit-check every time you use an N95 respirator

    c. You must wear the approved TB respirator (an N95 or a powered air purified respirator) every time you enter the room

    d. You may wear a surgical mask into the TB patient's room if you cannot find an approved TB respirator

    e. You must remove respirator outside of patient's room

9. You are receiving an emergency department admission with diagnosis of rule-out meningitis. Which of the following statements is *true*?

    a. Place the patient in a negative air pressure room until 24 hours after effective antibiotic therapy

    b. Place the patient in Droplet Precautions until 24 hours after effective antibiotic therapy and notify infection control

    c. Place the patient in Standard Precautions with a roommate

FIGURE 10.2 • SAMPLE INFECTION CONTROL COMPETENCY TEST (CONT.)

The following scenario applies to questions 10 and 11:

A 63-year-old male is admitted with a two-day history of diarrhea. The patient is developmentally disabled and is not capable of maintaining good hygiene. Significant history includes a recent admission for pneumonia and antibiotic therapy.

Fill in the blanks:

10. What communicable disease might this patient have? *Clostridium difficile*

11. What type of precautions would you implement? *Contact*

Circle the answer that applies.

12. Your patient is in Contact Precautions; which of the following does **NOT** reflect good infection control practices?

    a. Gown and glove every time you enter the patient's room to give patient care.

    b. Remove your gloves, gown and place in appropriate waste receptacle, wash hands then exit room. Wash hands.

    c. Remove gloves, wash hands, exit room. Remove gown and hang on isolation cart outside patient's room.

    d. Obtain Isolation Cart from Central Distribution.

    e. Place large green sign on patient's door.

Answer Key

1. c	7. a
2. c	8. d
3. c	9. b
4. a. True	10. (Fill in the blank)
5. b. False	11. (Fill in the blank)
6. a. True	12. c

Source: Reprinted with permission by Rosie Fardo.

FIGURE 10.3 • STANDARD AND TRANSMISSION-BASED PRECAUTIONS

Standard Precautions (S) is for all patients all the time. This includes appropriate hand washing and use of gloves, gowns, and eye protection.

Contact Precautions (C) is necessary when an illness is transmitted by direct contact. Recommendations include gloves, gown, and private room. Also, hand washing with an antimicrobial agent. Designate a blood pressure cuff and stethoscope for use only on that patient.

Droplet Precautions (D) is used for illnesses that are transmitted by large particle droplet and includes the use of a surgical mask when within 3 ft. of the patient

Airborne Precautions (A) is for illnesses transmitted by airborne nuclei and requires a specially ventilated negative pressure room and use of a N95 respirator or powered air purifying respirator

Common Disease/Organisms and Precautions Recommendations			
Standard (S)	**Contact (C)**	**Droplet (D)**	**Airborne (A)**

• AIDS/HIV
 	
• *E. coli* 0157:H7
  (C) if incontinent
 	
• Hepatitis A
  (C) if incontinent
 	
• Hepatitis B,C
 	
• Malaria
 	
• Streptococcal pneumonia
  (D) if infant
	• *Clostridium difficile*
	
	• Impetigo
	
	• Methicillan-resistant *Staphylococcus aureus*
	
	• Scabies
	
	• Vancomycin-resistant *Enterococci*
	
	• Empiric Precautions—clinical symptoms/syndromes warranting additional precautions pending confirmation of diagnosis
	
	• Diarrhea
	
	• History of multidrug-resistant organism
	
	• Skin or wound infection
	
	• Respiratory Infection in Children (croup or bronchiolitis)
		• Influenza
		
		• Meningitis
		  (Neisseria meningitidis, Haemophilus influenzae)
		
		• Mumps
		
		• Mycoplasma pneumonia
		
		• Parovirus B19
		
		• Pertussis
		
		• Rabies
		
		• *Streptococcal pharyngitis*
			• Positve for Acid-fast bacillus
			
			• Measles (rubeola)
			
			• Mycobacterium tuberculosis
			
			• Varicella
			  (also Contact)
			
			• Chicken pox, disseminated zoster

SPECIALIZED TRAINING

What about specialized training? This occurs often for the infection preventionist. An organism which the facility has never seen before is isolated from a new patient. An employee with an infectious disease may be allowed to work under very special conditions that require one-on-one education and training. The Joint Commission has also stated the need for training for physicians, contract workers such as construction workers, and volunteers.

This need is never so apparent than during an outbreak of infectious diseases. As the outbreak progresses and the facility tries to get control of the situation, much education is needed constantly to update staff members as well as leadership and physicians on the latest factual and accurate information (i.e., signs and symptoms of infection versus colonization, mode of transmission of the organism and isolation precautions, treatment, etc.) This may require special sessions for all three shifts of employees.

If the facility is Joint Commission–accredited, it must follow its National Patient Safety Goals and standards. At press, these cover:

- Complying with current World Health Organization hand hygiene guidelines or CDC hand hygiene guidelines.

- Identifying and treating all cases of unanticipated death or permanent loss of function related to healthcare-associated infections as sentinel events.

- Implementing best practices to prevent central line–associated bloodstream infections.

- Implementing best practices to prevent surgical site infections.

- Encouraging patients to be actively involved in their care (this involves patient/family education as well). See Figures 10.4 and 10.5 for examples of patient education pamphlets.

- Implementing evidence-based practices to prevent health care–associated infections due to multidrug-resistant organisms.

FIGURE 10.4 • SAMPLE INFECTION CONTROL EDUCATIONAL BROCHURE

There are types of diseases or infections that require us to use special precautions while providing care. These precautions are called **Contact Precautions.** We are using these precautions while caring for you. Your doctor and nurse can discuss this in more detail with you. This pamphlet is to help you understand what Contact Precautions are and why we use them.

Why do we use Contact Precautions?

When someone is known or suspected to be infected with certain germs that are highly contagious or harmful to our general patient population we place them in Contact Precautions. Examples of these are infections caused by antibiotic resistant germs, certain diarrheas, and certain types of wound infections. Doctors and nurses can carry these germs to other patients on their hands and clothing. Contact Precautions are used to prevent the spread of these infections to patients who are already ill.

What will be different?

- A Contact Precautions sign will be placed on your door so that visitors and caregivers will know to use special precautions.

- Hospital staff and doctors that enter the room will wear gloves. This will prevent them from carrying the germs out of the room.

- Hospital staff and doctors coming into your room may also be wearing a gown.

- All visitors entering the room must wear gloves and, when in contact with you or your environment, a gown.

- Everyone, staff and visitors, must wash his or her hands upon entering and leaving the room.

- If you are coughing frequently and productively, visitors and caregivers may wear a mask.

What about when I go home?

It is unlikely that you will need any special precautions after you are discharged. Remember the primary reason for Contact Precautions is to prevent the spread of infection in the hospital.

Hand washing is the key to preventing infection both at home and in the hospital. Use warm water and soap and wash for 10 to 15 seconds before eating, after toileting, after sneezing, and before and after providing care (such as changing a dressing) for your loved one.

No special care other than hot soapy water is needed for soiled laundry or eating utensils.

Remember, ask your doctor or nurse if you have any questions about your specific condition. If you would like to talk to someone from the Infection Control Department, ask your nurse to contact us.

Source: Reprinted with permission from Rosie Fardo.

FIGURE 10.5 • SAMPLE AIRBORNE PRECAUTIONS EDUCATIONAL BROCHURE

There are types of diseases or conditions that require us to use special precautions while providing care. One type of precaution we use is called **Airborne Precautions.** We are using these precautions while caring for you. Your doctor and nurse can discuss this in more detail with you. This pamphlet is to help you understand what Airborne Precautions are and why we use them.

Why do we use Airborne Precautions?

Airborne Precautions are used for patients known or suspected to have a disease that is spread by the airborne route. An example of such a disease is tuberculosis (TB). The airborne TB droplet is very small and can spread through the air current over a long distance. Even though we may not know for certain if you have TB, we must take precautions until your doctor can confirm the diagnosis. It may take several weeks until your tests are final. In the meantime, the law requires us to take precautions to prevent the spread of TB.

What will be different?

- An Airborne Precautions sign will be placed on your door so that visitors and caregivers will know to use special precautions.

- You will be required to stay in your room. If you must leave for a test, you will need to wear a mask while out of your room.

- Visitors and caregivers entering the room will be wearing a mask. The law requires employees entering the room of a patient with suspected or confirmed TB to wear a special mask. This will look different than the mask worn by your visitors.

- The door to your room must remain closed.

- Friends or family with chronic illnesses should consider waiting to visit until you have recovered.

How long will precautions be in place?

You will need to stay in Airborne Precautions until your doctor determines that you do not have TB or can no longer spread TB. If it is determined that you do have TB, your local TB Control will work with you at discharge to determine what kind of precautions you need to take at home.

How can you help?

- The TB germ is spread whenever an infected person sneezes, talks, coughs, or sings. Always cover your mouth and nose when sneezing or coughing.

- Wash your hands, often and well.

- If it is determined that you do have TB, it is very important that you take your medicine as prescribed by your doctor.

- *Remember,* ask your doctor or nurse if you have any questions about your condition. If you would like to talk with someone from the Infection Control Department, ask your nurse to contact us.

Source: Reprinted with permission from Rosie Fardo.

To remain current on the latest infectious diseases and trends in infection prevention, the IP must read constantly, be an active member of Association for Professionals in Infection Control and Epidemiology (APIC), and receive continual updates on infection prevention and control topics. Our national association, APIC, has wonderful educational opportunities and so will your state or chapter. Not only can you avail yourself of the knowledge of IPs who have been in the trenches, but you can begin to build a wonderful network for resources of other IPs struggling with similar issues. Who knows, you may even make the decision to become certified in your field!

CONCLUSION

The health and education of employees is really the other half of an active, effective infection prevention and control program focusing on the facility's patients. Employees are our greatest resource in the care of our patients.

REFERENCES

1. W.E. Scheckler, et al., "Requirements for Infrastructure and Essential Activities of Infection Control and Epidemiology in Hospitals: A Consensus Panel Report," *Infection Control and Hospital Epidemiology* 19.1 (1998): 114–124.

2. "Guideline for Infection Control in Health Care Personnel, 1998," Centers for Disease Control and Prevention, *www.cdc.gov.*

3. "Recommended Adult Immunization Schedule: United States, 2009," *Morbidity and Mortality Weekly Report* 57.53: 2008.

4. "Guideline for Infection Control in Health Care Personnel, 1998," Centers for Disease Control and Prevention, *www.cdc.gov.*

5. Ibid.

6. "Centers for Disease Control and Prevention Updated U.S. Public Health Service Guidelines for the Management of Occupational Exposures to HBV, HCV, and HIV and Recommendations for Postexposure Prophylaxis," *Morbidity and Mortality Weekly Report Recommendations and Reports* 50 (RR-11) (2001): 1–52.

7. "Guideline for Infection Control in Health Care Personnel, 1998," Centers for Disease Control and Prevention, *www.cdc.gov.*

8. K.K. Hoffman, E.P. Clontz, "Education Of Healthcare Workers In The Prevention Of Healthcare–Associated Infections," *Hospital Epidemiology and Infection Control* (Philadelphia, PA, Lippincott Williams and Wilkins, 2004), 1755-64.

9. H.A. Carr, P.L. Hinson, "Education and Training," APIC *Text of Infection Control and Epidemiology,* Second Edition, Washington, DC, APIC, 2005: 11-1—11-18.

FREE HEALTHCARE COMPLIANCE AND MANAGEMENT RESOURCES!

Need to control expenses yet stay current with critical issues?

Get timely help with FREE e-mail newsletters from HCPro, Inc., the leader in healthcare compliance education. Offering numerous free electronic publications covering a wide variety of essential topics, you'll find just the right e-newsletter to help you stay current, informed, and effective. All you have to do is sign up!

With your FREE subscriptions, you'll also receive the following:

- Timely information, to be read when convenient with your schedule

- Expert analysis you can count on

- Focused and relevant commentary

- Tips to make your daily tasks easier

And here's the best part—there's no further obligation—just a complimentary resource to help you get through your daily challenges.

It's easy. Visit *www.hcmarketplace.com/free/e-newsletters* to register for as many free e-newsletters as you'd like, and let us do the rest.

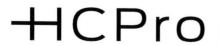

HCPro | Insight for healthcare compliance and management